Taking
NOTHING FOR
Granted

Taking
NOTHING FOR
Granted

Alastair
LYNCH

WITH PETER BLUCHER

A sportsman's
fight against
Chronic Fatigue
Syndrome

Harper*Sports*
An imprint of HarperCollins*Publishers*

Harper*Sports*
An imprint of HarperCollins*Publishers*

First published in Australia in 2005
This edition published in 2008
by HarperCollins*Publishers*, Australia Pty Limited
ABN 36 009 913 517
www.harpercollins.com.au

HarperCollins*Publishers*
25 Ryde Road, Pymble, Sydney NSW 2073, Australia
31 View Road, Glenfield, Auckland 10, New Zealand
1–A, Hamilton House, Connaught Place, New Delhi – 110 001, India
77–85 Fulham Palace Road, London W6 8JB, United Kingdom
2 Bloor Street East, 20th Floor, Toronto, Ontario M4W 1A8, Canada
10 East 53rd Street, New York NY 10022, USA

National Library of Australia Cataloguing-in-publication data:

Lynch, Alastair.
    Taking nothing for granted: a sportsman's fight against
    chronic fatigue syndrome / Alastair Lynch with Peter Blucher.
    Pymble, NSW: HarperCollins, 2008
    ISBN 978 0 7322 8811 2 (pbk.)
    Lynch, Alastair.
    Chronic fatigue syndrome – Patients – Australia.
    Australian football players – Biography.
    Blucher, Peter.
362.19604780092

Front cover image: Letchford Photography. Back cover image: Getty Images
Typeset in 11/18pt Goudy by Kirby Jones

To Peta,
Madison, Tom and Claudia

FOREWORD

BY PAUL ROOS

At the end of 1993 Alastair Lynch was, in my opinion, the most valuable player in the AFL. He could kick seven goals at full forward one day and the next day go to fullback to play on the best in the business, like Tony Lockett and Jason Dunstall. He was a champion, certainly among the best three players in the game, and such was his versatility that I wouldn't have traded him for Wayne Carey, widely regarded as the greatest player of all time.

It's inconceivable that within 12 months Lynchy was sleeping 18 hours a day. He had an illness which nobody could properly diagnose, let alone cure. The frustration and uncertainty of it all was horrendous. Football wasn't a consideration. It had become a fight for quality of life.

Now, more than a decade later, he's a retired triple-premiership player who will be remembered as one of the all-time greats. And, I'm happy to say, one of my great mates.

This is his story. But it is much more than the story of a champion footballer. It is the story of a man who gave meaning to a condition which most Australians had never heard of — chronic fatigue syndrome (CFS). He overcame this serious illness to not only fulfil his own dreams but provide an inspiration to tens of thousands of Australians; a reason for CFS-sufferers to believe they, too, could beat this shocking condition.

I met Lynchy in the summer of 1987–88 when he arrived at Fitzroy Football Club as a tall, skinny teenager from Hobart. He was more an athlete than a footballer but quickly he became both. For six years he was a Fitzroy teammate, and in his last year with the club in 1993 he was awesome.

I know how difficult it was for him to leave Fitzroy for Brisbane because he knew what a precarious position the club was in. There was enormous pressure on him to stay and he didn't want to let anyone down, but Fitzroy were already dying a slow death as a separate entity. Even though I was Fitzroy captain at the time, I was 100 per cent behind his decision to leave, and so were his senior teammates. We didn't want him to go but deep down we knew he had to look after himself and his future. It was too late for blind, unrequited loyalty when he had the opportunity to set himself up for life.

It was a tragedy that through his illness Brisbane were denied the services of Alastair Lynch in his prime. Who knows what he might have achieved had he not been sick? Maybe a Brownlow Medal, four or five club championships and a couple of 100-goal seasons. Nothing was beyond his capabilities.

But would he have played in three premiership sides if he'd not been sick? Who knows? Maybe his illness and 12 months out of football in 1995 actually prolonged his career. By necessity, he returned a different yet equally valuable player. He wasn't able to punish his body as most footballers do and this prolonged his career, allowing him to play several years beyond normal retirement age. And how well he played. Through the Brisbane Lions' triple premiership era of 2001–02–03 he was as important as any member of arguably the best side of all time.

Football owes Lynchy a huge debt. He played a massive role in developing the game in Queensland in the same way

Tony Lockett helped spread the football gospel in New South Wales. Like 'Plugger', he was such a strong individual. Fans love a big, aggressive player who has a real presence about him and kicks goals. It's a skill unique to AFL football and he captured the imagination of the football public.

Aside from my own football memories, the 2001 grand final, when Lynchy and the Brisbane Lions made history as the first team from a so-called developing state to win the AFL premiership, was my favourite. To be there on the sideline, to walk onto the ground and offer my congratulations, and to see him receive his premiership medallion, was such a powerful moment.

Quite simply, he deserved it. He's the most humble and unassuming person you'll meet. A loyal and generous friend, fantastic husband and devoted family man, he and his wife, Peta, had been to hell and back, and a change of fortune was long overdue.

To know the shocking illness Lynchy went through to savour the ultimate football triumph was incredible. Yet I don't fully understand it — it seems nobody really does. That's the nature of CFS. It's a terrible condition which strikes at random and confines normal, healthy people to bed for days, weeks and even months on end. And nobody knows why.

Through his sporting profile, Lynchy became the flagship for CFS sufferers in Australia. It wasn't a role he would ever pursue, because self-promotion simply isn't his go. I almost had to drag the details of his illness out of him, and this book tells many more.

He hesitated long and hard before agreeing to commit private and personal details of his remarkable tale to print because he's just not that sort of person. But in the end the opportunity to help CFS sufferers overruled his reluctance.

I'm pleased it did and proud to have been asked to write this foreword. For this is a book of true courage and inspiration. Of a person who, despite the extraordinary intervention of a truly shocking illness, never lost his most precious quality of being one outstanding human being. Well done mate.

Paul Roos

Contents

Acknowledgments

Chronic fatigue syndrome is something I wouldn't wish upon my worst enemy. It's an illness which struck me in the prime of my sporting life and robbed me of virtually 12 months of football, and affected the remainder of my career. There was no escape. It took my health and turned my life upside down. But, 10 years on, after an often difficult fight full of ups and downs I'm proud to say that I have beaten it — at least so that I can jump out of bed looking forward to the day ahead.

That would not have been possible without the support of countless hundreds of people. And while I have dedicated this book to my wife Peta and my children Madison, Tom and Claudia, the most important people in my life, I also want to acknowledge collectively so many others who have helped along the way. Not just during my CFS years but throughout my entire life.

I'm fortunate to have a wonderfully loyal, generous and supportive group of family and close friends. They are too numerous to mention individually here but they know who they are — thank you one and all.

Also, to the Fitzroy and Brisbane football clubs. I could not have chosen two better footballing 'homes'. Win or lose, the people were fantastic through my 17 years in the AFL. Players, coaches, administrators, sponsors and support staff members alike, they went out of their way to help make my job of trying to get a kick that much easier. Likewise, at the Hobart and Wynyard football clubs, where I played before joining the AFL. There's something about football people that makes them special.

But football is about more than just those on the inside. The supporters live and breathe the game and were just fantastic to me. To the Fitzroy people, sorry for leaving. And to the Brisbane people, thanks for making me and my family feel so welcome. Collectively, you make a sensational team. I appreciate enormously the support of every one of you, and I hope the good times we shared in the last few years of my career repaid the debt of gratitude that all players owe their loyal band of fans.

That I was able to enjoy the excitement and satisfaction of three AFL premierships in the years after I thought my career was over was due largely to the medical people who eventually worked out what was wrong with me, and helped me get on top of it. Thank you.

A special thanks to my good mate Paul Roos, who wrote the generous foreword for this book, and whose support has never wavered. Also, to those friends and associates who gave of their time and insight so willingly to assist this project.

I also thank Peter Blucher, with whom I have written *Taking Nothing for Granted*. It was a task I would not have undertaken without his support, advice, direction and encouragement. And, at times, his persuasive and persistent 'we've got to get it done'. To have a friend who had seen from close quarters the CFS chapter of my life and shared the football success was good; that he could help write my story was even better.

Finally, I want to thank each and every CFS sufferer with whom I have ever had any association. Those who offered their help to me, and those who appreciated the help I tried to offer them. Each in their own way is an inspiration.

I feel for anyone struck down by illness; for CFS sufferers I encourage each and every one of you to be patient and listen to, and learn about your body. Do the things that work for you, avoid the things that don't. In the end you can beat it. This book is for every chronic fatigue sufferer.

Thank you and good luck.

Alastair Lynch

1

THE DEFINING MOMENT

At 5.13pm at the MCG on Saturday, 29 September 2001, the siren sounded to end the AFL grand final. We had won. I had the ball in my hands. I thrust it skywards and stood still with a silly grin on my face. It is every kid's dream. A fantasy come true, right down to the very last detail. Time stood still — for I don't know how long — as a myriad of thoughts raced through my head.

It's an unbelievable and unexplainable adrenaline rush as your mind races from one picture to another. From the little kid kicking the footy in the backyard dreaming of winning an AFL grand final to the thousands of hours of hard slog, all done for one reason: this very moment.

You think of the mates with whom you've shared your greatest triumph, and without whom you would be just another dreamer — mates who have stood beside you through so much, and who are now running amok beside you as they live this incredible moment in their own way.

In this short moment of solitary reflection amid a packed stadium, in front of a worldwide television audience of millions, my mind raced over the days when I was convinced I'd never make it, caught as I was in the relentless grasp of chronic fatigue syndrome (CFS). I was sleeping 18 hours a day and wanting to sleep even more. And I thought about the one person without whom I would not possibly have made it: my wife Peta.

There were so many crises, like the time I'd been charged by the AFL with taking a prohibited substance. What I had taken was simply part of a prescribed medication package for CFS, yet the league was effectively branding me a drug cheat. How grateful I was, now, that my name had been cleared.

My mind even flashed back to three weeks earlier, to the qualifying final against Port Adelaide, when I'd been reported for striking Power fullback Darryl Wakelin. We'd won that match, which put us just one game away from the grand final; the prospect of a two-match suspension, which would have ruled me out of the premiership decider, had been mortifying.

But from mortification to triumph. As the grand final time clock ticked on I had wandered away from my customary position at full forward. I found myself up on centre wing, in front of the Great Southern Stand. This was unusual. I never ventured far from the goal square. Why did I do it? I don't know. Teammate Brad Scott had the footy at halfback. He kicked it to me and I took a mark. As I looked at our goal I could see the time clock on the scoreboard at the Punt Road end of the ground in the background. It read 30-something minutes. We were 27 points up, and I realised there couldn't be long to go. Immediately, the siren went.

Chris Scott was the nearest Lions player. We enjoyed an embrace which, if it hadn't been such a special football moment, might have started people wondering. The umpire asked for the ball. 'You're not serious, are you?' I replied. But he was. It was AFL regulations that one of the umpires takes the ball from the ground, he explained. So, much to the disgust of teammates nearby, I handed it over. The umpire promised to get it back to me afterwards but I doubted I'd ever see it again. Who cared?

It was one of eight footballs made especially for the grand final, with grand final and team branding. In this game they used only four, one in each quarter — first, it was a fine day, and second, no balls were lost in the crowd. And yes, I did get one. The following year the Lions presented me with one of the four balls that had not been used. It wasn't quite the same, but it had been signed by the umpires to authenticate it, so it's still a very special keepsake of a very special moment. I really appreciated the club's generosity.

Slowly the players, dotted all over the ground when the siren sounded, gathered in the middle. It was pandemonium. For several minutes, maybe longer, it could have been 4am on the dance floor of a nightclub. Not that I really knew what 4am on a nightclub dance floor was like, but it was total chaos here at the ground. Everyone was hugging everyone else, unable to comprehend what we'd achieved. Two words were repeated time and again almost as if to make sure they were really true. 'We won!'

I even bumped into one of my best mates, Paul Roos, who was masquerading as a boundary reporter for grand final telecasters Channel Seven. I was really pleased to see him. He'd been such a mentor and such a good friend. It didn't strike me at the time, but I remembered later that Roosy had played 269 games at Fitzroy (between 1982 and 1994) without reaching a grand final, and in 1996 had lost the only premiership decider he played during his

87 games with Sydney (from 1995 to 1998). He was genuinely thrilled that I'd finally achieved the ultimate in football. I suppose that's another reason why premierships are so special: even people like Roos, one of the absolute greats of the game, sometimes miss out. Individually you can be the best, but that doesn't guarantee team success.

Shaun Hart received the Norm Smith Medal for the best player in the grand final from ex-Essendon star Jack Clarke. That was an unforgettable moment in itself. Never has there been a more selfless person play AFL football — Harty is a proud and wonderful Christian who cares more about others than about himself. He was a deserving winner.

Then Clarke and triple Brownlow medallist Ian Stewart presented premiership medallions to each player individually. In jumper number order we floated up onto the stage to receive that special memento. I was rapt to get mine from Stewart, a former St Kilda and Richmond champion and a fellow Tasmanian.

Master of Ceremonies Craig Willis, an old mate of mine from Fitzroy days, called out the names. 'No. 2 — Chris Johnson,' he said. He skipped No. 3. Michael Voss was the captain. He would be last. 'No. 4 — Craig McRae.' Then Brad Scott, Luke Power, Tim Notting, Marcus Ashcroft and yours truly. Then Jason Akermanis,

Martin Pike, Mal Michael, Jonathan Brown, Simon Black, Chris Scott, Justin Leppitsch, Clark Keating, Robbie Copeland, Hart, Darryl White, Daniel Bradshaw, Beau McDonald and Nigel Lappin. And finally Voss.

Leigh Matthews received the Jock McHale Medal from Robbie McHale, the great grand-daughter of the legendary Collingwood coach after whom the medal for the premiership coach was named. And then Stewart presented the premiership cup to captain Vossy and Leigh. The players invaded the stage. Champagne corks popped wildly. There was a rushed team photograph with the cup and then the victory lap. How sweet it was. How long it took. And how many familiar faces did I see as we walked ever so slowly around the inside of the fence!

The emotion among the supporters was little different from that of the players. Many from the Fitzroy side of the Brisbane–Fitzroy merger, which had formed the Brisbane Lions in 1997, had waited since their last flag, in 1944, to savour premiership glory. And for the Brisbane-ites it was an altogether new experience. They'd never tasted the sweetest taste of all.

This was the day the marriage of the two clubs was consummated. It was the first merger in AFL history, and while not always sweet and harmonious, it was always the right thing for both parties. The merger had been perfect for me because it brought together my two clubs: Fitzroy, where I'd played from 1988 to 1993, and Brisbane, where I'd played since 1994.

About a third of the way around the lap of honour I found Peta, who, with Donna Voss, had hurried down to the fence from the players' enclosure. They'd sat there and lived every kick and every goal. That prolonged embrace with my wife was special — and was much better than the one with Chris Scott in the first few seconds after the siren!

Peta had been through it all. She'd been stronger than any woman had a right to be. Like all the wives and girlfriends, she'd put up with the endless demands of a coach and a football operation that accepted only absolute commitment. Unlike her counterparts, Pete had also been a pivotal part of our fight against CFS. And we'd won.

I put my premiership medal around her neck. It was my way of saying thank you. The symbol of football achievement which meant so much to me was with her as I rejoined the lap of honour. More hugs. More handshakes. More slaps on the back. It seemed endless.

There were also members of the Lions playing group who hadn't played in the grand final: the emergency trio of Matthew Kennedy, Des Headland and Aaron Shattock, plus Craig Bolton and Dylan McLaren. They probably had mixed emotions, but outwardly, at least, they were relishing the moment. They were a real part of it, too, because they had done the hard work throughout the long campaign just like the rest of us.

Even the Essendon cheer squad had some kind words before we finally reached the players' race that led to the dressing rooms. I was the last player to leave the ground. And I had the cup. It made a photograph that was splashed all over the papers — one I'll long treasure.

Inside we gathered one last time in the coach's room. Leigh Matthews told us how proud he was of the team and reminded us to be humble in victory. 'Just because you've won, don't feel you need to celebrate like fools,' he told us. 'Don't be silly — just enjoy it.' Good advice and important, too, but I don't think it was necessary. The quality of the Brisbane Lions team wasn't just in how they played. This was one very special group of people. They didn't have to be told to be gracious winners; still this was a coach who left nothing to chance.

And then, standing in a tight circle in a tiny room deep in the bowels of the Olympic Stand at the MCG, we shared a team-only moment. Passing the champagne-filled cup around, each of us spoke about the player next to us and what he meant to us. It was a fitting finale to the formal team-only part of the celebrations. I'll never forget it — if only I could remember what was said! At 33, I was the oldest member of our team, which is my only excuse. Whether I remember the words or not, though, the moment was special.

In the rooms outside we found a lot of familiar faces: ex-club mates Andrew Bews, Andy Gowers, Richard Champion, Matthew Campbell and Trent Bartlett, for a start. Big 'Bart', a fellow Tasmanian, was miffed. He'd backed me to kick the first goal and was filthy that I'd missed a set shot in the first few minutes. 'Bart, I missed that one, but I still kicked the first one,' I told him. Too late; he'd thrown the ticket away in disgust.

If that moment which I shared with the people who matter most to me could have lasted forever I would have been the happiest person on earth. There is no adequate description for the feeling: it's an extraordinary mix of elation and disbelief, pride and pleasure, vindication and contentment. And of absolute fulfilment.

I could have retired right there and then and been totally satisfied. Unbelievably, it was here.

*   *   *

As much as I treasured my bond with my football family, I also felt a deep sense of delight because of the message my role in the Lions' success would send to another group for whom I had great empathy: the chronic fatigue syndrome (CFS) family.

Six years earlier I had been a member of that group, a group that now numbers about 150,000 Australians — people whose quality of life has been inexplicably stolen by an illness which a large portion of the medical fraternity still insist doesn't exist.

That was me in 1995. I missed virtually the entire AFL season, though football was the furthest thing from my mind. I didn't care about football; I just wanted my health back. I wanted to be able to get out of bed in the morning feeling refreshed and enthusiastic about the day ahead. To be able to do what normal people do without shocking headaches — and without feeling utterly helpless and massively frustrated because nobody could tell me when I'd get better.

Because of my public profile, I'd unwittingly become something of a flagship for CFS sufferers in Australia. It wasn't something I wanted, or something I felt comfortable with, initially. But as time wore on and I found a way back to football at the highest level, I realised that I was providing hope for other CFS patients.

Over the years I've received thousands of letters, emails, faxes and phone calls from people who have CFS and are desperately looking for advice. I've tried one way or another to help as many as I can, but it hasn't been easy and hasn't always been possible. It would have been a full-time job, and then some.

I will be really pleased if my being able to resume playing football has given just one person a little inspiration. I guess it is proof, if you like, that there is life after CFS and that you can overcome this condition.

That is the only reason I agreed to write this book. I hope that by writing about my ongoing battle with CFS, detailing how it affected my life as a professional footballer, and the countless lessons I've learned along the way, I might be able to help fellow CFS sufferers.

There is rarely a day that goes by without me thinking about CFS, and about how fortunate I've been to be able to overcome the condition sufficiently to live a normal life. I can now share with my wife Peta and children Madison, Tom and Claudia the sort of everyday things which everyday people too often take for granted.

Grand final day 2001 was no different. And amid the excitement and celebrations, I also felt a sense of pride that maybe, just maybe, my football achievements would help long-time CFS victims keep fighting and keep hoping.

It is a fight that can be won. I don't know if I've totally shed myself of CFS, because I've never been brave enough to abandon the strict lifestyle protocols and disciplines that have been my daily routine from the time I became ill. I'll probably never know, because I'll never do anything to jeopardise my quality of life.

But I can promise CFS sufferers that you can overcome the symptoms enough to live a normal life; to play AFL football, even. After all, there I was on grand final day 2001, living testimony that it can be done.

2

THE EARLY DAYS

As the father of three children I live by the creed that my main responsibility in life, in partnership with my wife Peta, is to provide Madison, Tom and Claudia with as many different experiences and opportunities as possible. To help them learn as many lessons as they can; to understand the difference between right and wrong; to appreciate qualities like fairness, honesty and integrity; and to recognise the invaluable worth of friendship, health and happiness. To help prepare them for adulthood, so that when they have to make their own decisions and fend for themselves they will have a good foundation on which to base their adult lives.

From the moment they were born, the children have been the most important thing in my life — along with my wife. They are the reason I get out of bed with a zest for life every day, and go to bed at night with a degree of satisfaction and contentment.

So, as I recall my own childhood, it's interesting to reflect on how different episodes were important learning experiences. How the values I try to live by as an adult and parent were formed. How sport became such a useful tool for someone who didn't exactly excel in the classroom. And how fortunate I was to be born to loving parents who took on the same obligations I now try to fulfil with my own family. Even if there were a few unavoidable and unfortunate hiccups along the way.

I was born on 19 June 1968 in Burnie, the fourth-biggest town in Tasmania behind Hobart, Launceston and Devonport; it has a population of about 20,000. My father, Graeme, was a born-and-bred Burnie-ite, if such a word exists. After playing under-age football and hockey for Tasmania, he became a clerk with the Burnie Council and continued sport at a senior level. He split his sporting year between playing ruck-rover and half forward with the Burnie Tigers, as they were then known, then the Wynyard Cats, and opening the batting for the Burnie Cricket Club (later Wynyard). He had one year in the Tasmanian Football League with Glenorchy, and all up played 197 games before retiring at age 27 and going coaching at nearby Smithton. He even had a trial with Richmond. He went across to Melbourne for three weeks in 1963, and did 13 weeks pre-season in 1964. He played a few practice matches, but couldn't get a clearance from Burnie. Or at least that's what he told us.

His great claim to fame was playing at full forward in a Tasmanian Under 14 side that competed in an Australian carnival at the Gabba in Brisbane in 1959. Not because he was a superstar, but because on the wing in the same side was Peter Hudson, who was to kick 727 goals in 129 AFL games for Hawthorn and become one of the greatest full forwards of all time. Barry Lawrence, later to captain St Kilda and father a son, Steven, with whom I would play in Brisbane, was also in the Tasmanian side. Future Richmond champion Billy Barrot, and Carl Ditterich, later a star with St Kilda and Melbourne, played in the same carnival for Victoria.

My mother Marjorie was from Barkingside, Ilford, Essex, in the south of England. She emigrated as a 12-year-old to Australia when her parents decided to follow her father's parents Down Under. They sailed on the *Strathaird*, a big P&O liner, and lived at Kingston

Beach, south of Hobart, before moving north to Blythe Heads, 5km outside Burnie. She was a keen sports follower, too. She was a good swimmer, played basketball, did some running, and also used to own a horse.

I was named after Alistair Lord, the 1962 Brownlow medallist and Geelong's 1963 premiership centreman. He was appointed Burnie coach in 1965 but didn't last too long before he was lured back to Geelong to continue what was an outstanding AFL career. Lord was what my dad describes as 'such a good bloke', even if they did spell my first name slightly differently from his. Was it done by design or accident? It depends who you ask.

I was the oldest of three Lynch boys. Vaughan was 21 months younger than me, and Manuel 12 months younger again. Our first home was a two-storey brick place on a block of land sloping up from the road in Grandview Avenue, Burnie. We spent a lot of time at West Park, where Dad played footy. There were always plenty of kids around and we split our time between rock fights behind the little grandstand, the battle to get the footy after someone kicked a goal, and trying to con the ladies in the canteen into giving us free hotdogs.

I was five when we moved to Wynyard in 1973 after Dad transferred in the council, and it was there that I first started playing sport. Wynyard only had about 5000 people, but they just loved their sport and have produced more than their share of stars. In football alone there have been plenty — Hawthorn's Colin Robertson, winner of the 1983 Norm Smith Medal; Geelong 200-gamer Robert 'Scratcher' Neal; Richmond 100-gamer and Fremantle captain Chris Bond; Paul Williams, a dual Best & Fairest winner at Sydney after time at Collingwood; and Footscray/Fitzroy star Simon Atkins and his twin brother Paul, who played at Sydney. We'd even claim Michael and Brendon Gale, who lived in the municipality of Wynyard before playing at Fitzroy and Richmond respectively; and Ben Buckley, a North Melbourne vice-captain who was from nearby Smithton but lived at a hostel in Wynyard when he went to school. He later became a marketing heavyweight with the AFL.

Wynyard was also home to Tasmanian cricketers Jamie Cox and Dene Hills; and Carla Boyd, an Australian basketball representative, was our neighbour in Austin Street. There was a vacant lot between our house and the Boyds' house, with only a milk storage shed on it, so that was always a good playground if we didn't feel like making the short trek to the footy ground at the end of the street. It was at the Boyd house that I first sampled Dad's beer.

Shocking stuff. Enough to put me off for a lot of years, but sadly it wasn't terminal.

Wynyard Primary School was more about catching up with my mates than schoolwork. I was never one to miss school because there was always a game of cricket or soccer to be had, but I wasn't a great scholar. My report cards were pretty consistent — 'If Alastair would apply himself . . .'

I believe sport is a fantastic learning tool itself. First and foremost, it teaches you about being part of a team, and that is something that can be applied to just about everything you do later in life. If you can't work with others you can't work. Even when you're a beginner, sport teaches you about many important things: discipline, training, helping others, enjoying the success of others, and how to win and lose.

My first game of footy was when I was six, playing for the Green Hornets in the mini-league at Wynyard Showgrounds. It wasn't until I was 15 that football really took over from soccer as my preferred winter sport. I played Under 17s and Under 19s with the Wynyard Cats, who wore a Carlton-style jumper with WFC on the front, before switching to the Geelong uniform and back again.

I was elected captain of the Under 17s by the players, but only as a joke — I wasn't very good. So after I tossed the coin in my first game at Les Clark Oval, Cooee, I took up my position on the bench. I was lucky to even get in the side. The coach, Doug Bachelor, knew what he was doing.

The following year we won the 1985 North-West Football Union Under 19s premiership. I was no longer captain, but it was a pretty handy team. It included Chris Bond, later to play at Carlton, Richmond and Fremantle; and Jamie Cox, who was drafted by Essendon before deciding to concentrate on cricket. Also claimed from the Wynyard Under 19s by AFL clubs, either via the draft or the old Form Four interstate recruiting process, were Andrew Reynolds (Essendon), Andrew Herring (Carlton) and Michael Neal (Geelong). The coach of that team was Wally Scott.

One day about mid-season, at Latrobe, after playing a full game in the Under 19s, the Reserves were short so I doubled up. It was the sort of thing that used to happen occasionally in small country towns, when player numbers were limited and work commitments would occasionally intervene to reduce the numbers even further. Fifteen minutes into the Reserves game I took a mark on the lead, and as I spun around to look at the goals I hurt my ankle. It was originally diagnosed as a bad sprain, but four weeks later, when it had shown little sign of improvement, it was found to have two fractures. My ankle was put in plaster and that was football for the year. Or so I thought. On the Tuesday night of Under 19s grand final week I was watching the boys train and thought to myself, I wouldn't mind playing. So I cut the plaster off, trained on the Thursday night, to prove I could at least run, and played against Cooee at West Park Oval on the Saturday. I was no great contributor playing on and off the bench, but I had a premiership medal, and it would be a long, long time before I had another.

As a young kid I was pretty average in size; it was only when I got to 15 or 16 that I started to shoot up. So in summer I was a wicket-keeper — or a keeper/batsman, I liked to think. I looked very classy with the bat and played some of the all-time great innings in the nets, but I rarely produced in the middle. Cox, later to become a Tasmanian stalwart and one of the best cricketers never to play for Australia, was a year younger than me but he was so good that he always played out of his age group. Hills was a year younger again, so I didn't play with him until we got to the seniors.

I was 16 when I was promoted from A Reserve to A Grade in 1984, and by that time I was a fast bowler who tended to bowl a bit on the short side. I really loved cricket — but only when we were fielding. Batting invariably meant sitting around watching, and when I did get a hit, I never lasted long. Still, in 1985 I was invited to do winter training with the Tasmanian Sheffield Shield squad. They used to split their time between Hobart, Launceston and Devonport, and on the recommendation of Les Allen, the Wynyard coach and Tasmania's former backup keeper to Roger Woolley, I got a call from Graham Mansfield. He was the state coach and a lovely bloke. It was all arranged for me to go to Devonport, but I'd broken my ankle the weekend before.

My early sporting life had gone pretty much according to plan. I loved my footy and I loved my cricket. But things hadn't gone quite so smoothly at home. My parents had split up when I was in Year 4. To this day I don't know why. I've never asked, and frankly I don't need to know. It has just made me value my own marriage and family life even more, if that's possible. Mum and Dad were never anything but sensational to me, giving me all the love and support I could ever have wanted.

I was 10 and just starting to enjoy time with my brothers in that typical brotherly love–hate way when we were separated. I was living with Dad in Wynyard while Vaughan and Manuel lived with Mum in Launceston,

200km — two hours — away. That was a long way in Tasmania in those days, and we only saw each other a handful of times a year.

After that I moved around a bit. I completed Year 5 in Wynyard then I did Year 6 at Somerset Primary School, and Year 7 at St Patrick's College in Launceston, while I lived with Mum for a year. But as much as I loved living with Mum and my brothers, it meant Dad was by himself. That didn't seem fair, so I returned to Somerset, a small town outside Burnie, and did Years 8–10 at Burnie High School.

In 1984–85 I was enrolled to do matriculation, Years 11 and 12, at Hellyer College while living in Wynyard with Dad and his second wife, Mollie, and her three sons Robbie, Danny and Steven, who have all become good friends. The boys' older sister Vicki had already married and left home. Dad was working in industrial relations with the King River Dam Hydro-Electric Scheme at Queenstown. It was 200km south on the west coast and he only came home on weekends. Two-thirds of the way through Year 11 I accepted a job as a geology assistant on the King River scheme, the alternative to the Gordon Below Franklin Hydro-Electric Scheme, which had been abandoned due to world heritage considerations. I was allowed to complete my Year 11 exams, but that was the end of my formal education. My final report said something like, 'If Alastair applied himself . . .'

At the time I didn't have any regrets about not completing school, but with the benefit of 20 years in the real world, I'd now say to any youngster, 'Make sure you finish your education.' Or at least get some training behind you. If it's not a tertiary qualification, make it a trade. Life has become too competitive not to at least try to give yourself a good solid start.

At the time I was happy to be out in the workforce earning $150 a week. I was 16 and living in single man's quarters with 650 others. They were prefab huts at a site known as 'Crotty' — which is now at the bottom of Lake Burbury. All you had was a bedroom and a small desk. You shared showers and toilets. There was no television reception, so they ran a video channel with a mixture of movies each night. A lot of the movies didn't seem to have much of a story line, though.

I was an assistant rock doctor. I hope this sounds technical: I worked with a nuclear densometer. This meant I'd walk along and hammer a giant steel rod into a road before it was sealed, to test the road's density. If the density wasn't right they'd have to dig it up and start again. Pretty demanding stuff, I promise you. I did that for 12 months from June 1984, going home to Wynyard on weekends to stay with family friends Joan and Barry Innes while I was playing cricket and football.

It was at Queenstown I got the best knock-back of my career. I thought I'd play football down there, rather than commute to Wynyard, but I was told I wouldn't make it. And aren't I happy about that! Because at Queenstown they played on a gravel oval, with a concrete cricket pitch in the middle, and a bitumen bike track around the outside. And nothing else. Not a blade of grass. And it wasn't just heavy sand. It was real gravel. Possibly a football oval that was unique world-wide.

Dad and Mollie moved permanently to Queenstown in 1984, so I lived with my grandparents, Bert and Ethel Lynch, in Burnie after I accepted my second job — shift work in a timber mill in Somerset. This was a pretty complex job, too. I'd feed freshly sliced sheets of veneer, each about 2m long, into a dryer. I worked with big John 'Frog' Newman. All 140kg of him. He was a fitter and turner, and a legendary local footballer. Other workmates were Under 19s teammates Peter Alderson and Leigh Gregory, who later played football on the Gold Coast and was a volunteer statistician for a game I played at Carrara many years later with Fitzroy. If we felt the timber mill job was getting too taxing, we'd deliberately fray the end of one of the sheets of veneer so it would jam the rollers on the dryer and they'd have to shut the machine down to fix the problem. That's when 'Frog' came in. We'd go and find the big man, explain the problem and he'd reply with the standard question: 'How long do you want off?' Usually 30 minutes was good.

There was a downside to the job — apart from the fact that it was about as boring as watching paint dry — you couldn't help but get a wet veneer sap on your hands, and as soon as you touched metal it caused your hands to turn black. There was no washing it off. You just had to work it off the following day. I did my best to avoid it, because it was pretty ugly, but sometimes there was no getting it off. Like the day just before Christmas 1985, when I was to make what would be a life-changing trip to Hobart.

I was 17 and armed with a driver's licence but no car. I was still rebuilding my 1969 Corolla station wagon after a little encounter with Mt Black on the way to work one morning. I spent a lot of time at the home of my good mate Darren 'Greasy' Smith, a junior teammate. He was a trained mechanic and, with Mick Foster, we used to cruise around in his beat-up old Kombi van. He also happened to have a car similar to mine. It had a bad ding in the back end and was undrivable, so we took the left front panel off it, even though it was orange, and put it on my white car. A work of mechanical art if ever there was one. No wonder I didn't forge a career in that line of work.

There would have been plenty who suggested that my dad was optimistic in thinking I'd ever be any good at football. After all, I'd been to the western division trials for the northwest Tasmanian Under 17 side, a long way down from what was then the Teal Cup side, and I didn't even get a look in.

Still, Dad had arranged for me to visit his old Under 14 teammate Peter Hudson. Huddo was set to take over as coach of the Hobart Football Club in 1986 and Dad had asked him to give me a run. Huddo had also arranged a job interview for me with Westpac, through the Hobart captain, Scott Wade, a long-serving state rover and the previous Hobart coach, and now general manager of the Tasmanian Football League.

So, having worked the night shift, I met Mick Foster for the drive south. Now a member of the CIB in Devonport, he was then a boilermaker in Wynyard, and thought a couple of days in Hobart would be good. It was almost four hours to the state capital, and though I tried hard not to touch any metal, it was impossible not to.

When I arrived at the Brisbane Hotel, the resident hotel of the Hobart Football Club, all set to meet the legendary Peter Hudson in the lounge bar, my hands were jet black.

I was more than a little nervous. I was lucky Huddo was just as good a bloke as he was a footballer; otherwise it could have been soul-destroying. He made me feel right at ease and we had a good laugh about my black hands.

I didn't get the job at the bank — I don't think they believed my story about my hands — but Huddo looked after everything else. He organised some work for me at his own hotel, the Granada Tavern, and arranged for me to board with one of the staff members, Doreena Imlak. She lived in Mt Stuart, which was just around the corner from Huddo's place. So I went home for Christmas, packed up a few things, and headed back to Hobart to begin the next phase of my life.

On my first day as a Hobart resident I went to state Under 19 cricket practice. There, in the nets, I saw this blond little fella who batted quite nicely and bowled a few off-breaks and medium-pacers. Every time he'd beat the bat or hit the pads he'd appeal. A bit of a smart-arse, I thought, but he could play.

The next day I was off to pre-season training with Peter Hudson and the Hobart Football Club. And there he was again, the same little bloke, drilling 45m drop punts with his left foot and hitting the target every time. He could play football, too. It was Mathew Armstrong, later to become a long-time Fitzroy teammate and close friend, and now coach of the Tassie Devils in the VFL.

Armstrong played Under 19s cricket for Tasmania and was later chosen in the Tasmanian Sheffield Shield squad. He would have played for Tasmania, I'm sure, had his desire to play AFL football not been even stronger than his passion for cricket. I just played cricket with University in the City League. We played on turf wickets, but it was never anything more than a 50 over slogging session on a Saturday afternoon. I couldn't be bothered with the two-day games — they took up the whole of Saturday and Sunday. After all, I was in Hobart to play football. And learn about life.

Football under Huddo was a bit of a rude awakening. It was the first pre-season I'd done and it was pretty tough. Some of the runs on the road around the old TCA Oval on top of the Domain at Glebe were shockers. Speaking to some of the coach's ex-teammates, they'd say he never trained that hard, but he certainly flogged us. One week the closest thing to a skills session was doing 800m runs with a footy in our hand.

In my first senior practice match against Clarence I played on Greg Farquhar, a great Tassie player at the time. Ironically, I would also play on him in my last game in Hobart, when he got a two-week suspension for knocking me out. I ran around at centre half forward and did enough for Huddo to persist. I don't think I was very good, actually, but he'd gone to so much trouble for me he probably felt he had to give me every chance. If I hadn't had that personal relationship with him I doubt I would have been given as many chances. I might have been back working on the veneer production line.

But persist he did. He pushed me so hard, in fact, that sometimes I got a bit frustrated by the workload. After all, I was a kid from the northwest coast looking for a bit of fun in Hobart. Looking back now, though, I feel it was sensational of him, one of the legends of the game, to take such a personal interest in me. He was always out on the track, kicking his flat punts, and often he would put me up against teammate Wayne Fox, a long-time member of the Tasmanian side and the biggest and best full forward in the competition. Sometimes, even, Huddo would work one-on-one with me after training, and once he arranged a special session with Royce Hart, who was only the centre half forward in the AFL Team of the Century.

Off the track, too, he looked after me. I'd worked over the summer at his hotel, but after that he arranged a job for me as a ute driver, delivering spare parts for Repco. I often had dinner with Huddo and his wife Steph at their home. He'd even give me some extra pocket money by letting me mow his lawns. And when I'd finished we'd have a cold drink in the front yard and talk about life; about how you set yourself up; about how he'd worked hard to get his hotel behind him. And we'd talk about football. It was mind-blowing stuff. Here I was, a 17-year-old from nowhere enjoying the personal guidance of a guy whose goals-per-game average of 5.59 is the highest in AFL history. A guy who four times kicked 100-plus goals in a season, including an equal league record 150 in 1971, before a knee injury in Round 1 of 1972. And who, after retiring at the end of 1974, made a staggering comeback in 1977, aged 31, and then kicked his fifth ton and topped the league goal-kicking for a fourth time. He was like a second father to me. Just sensational. Words can't describe how much I appreciate his help. Suffice it to say that without him I would never have played AFL football.

In my early days in Hobart I boarded with Doreena in a two-bedroom unit at 1/1 Una Street, Mt Stuart. Doreena was a barmaid in the front bar at the Granada, Huddo's pub. I stayed with her for two years and she looked after me a treat. She gave me great support and guidance. I've not kept in touch with her, which is embarrassing. I must give her a call.

Hobart had two established forwards in 1986 — Wayne Fox and Carey Millhouse — so I was used as a floater. I played at centre half back, a bit on the wing, and on a flank at either end. It wasn't a bad side. It included Matty Armstrong, who later played 175 games with Fitzroy and North Melbourne, in the centre, and a young Paul Hudson, son of Peter, who played in a forward pocket. A future 242-game player at Hawthorn and the Western Bulldogs, he was 15 going on 16 and already played twice a day. He'd kick eight goals for Hutchins School in the morning and six in the afternoon for Hobart. We also had Andrew Lamprill, who later played 36 games at Melbourne, and Jamie Shanahan, who would play 162 games with St Kilda and Melbourne. We missed the finals, but somebody must have thought I did all right because I won the 1986 Tasmanian Football League (TFL) Rookie of the Year Award.

It seemed word had filtered across Bass Strait, too, because I had a few AFL talent scouts on my case. Arthur Wilson, Football Manager at Fitzroy, came down to Hobart twice, and even coach David Parkin saw me play at North Hobart Oval one day. I played up forward and kicked 2.5. Typical. I also had some calls from John Hook at Hawthorn and Graeme 'Gubby' Allan at Collingwood.

As a kid I'd barracked for Essendon, I don't know why. I didn't really have a hero, but Billy Duckworth was my favourite player. Ironically, in my first senior practice match for Fitzroy I played against Essendon at Windy Hill and Billy gave me a clip behind the ear. It made me realise they were serious about their footy in the big time.

After I moved to Hobart I established a strong rapport with Hawthorn via Huddo. I remember the great Peter Knights visiting Huddo in Hobart one time. And on the 1986 Hobart end-of-season trip we went to Melbourne to watch the Hawthorn–Carlton grand final. On the Thursday it was the Caulfield Races before we went to watch Hawthorn training at Glenferrie Oval. Huddo took me inside the inner sanctum. They treated me really well, but only because I was with the legend. Otherwise it would have been, 'What are you doing in here, son? Out the door.' But it was enough to really whet my appetite. To start the ambition burning. Never before had I desperately wanted to play football at the elite level, but all of a sudden it was there. And because I'd had this extra special treatment from Huddo and had met a few league players, it didn't seem quite as far away as in reality it was.

This was the first year of the national draft, when each AFL club would select five players from outside the League. There would be five rounds, each in the reverse finishing order of the 1986 season after competition newcomers Brisbane. So Brisbane had first pick each round, then wooden-spooners St Kilda would have second pick, Melbourne third, Richmond fourth, through until premiers Hawthorn closed out each round.

Draft day was 26 November 1986. Hawthorn and Collingwood overlooked me. The Hawks chose two Hobart boys — Darrin Pritchard (Sandy Bay) and Matthew Queen (Glenorchy) — plus Clayton Lamb (West Adelaide), Robin McKinnon (West Adelaide) and Tony Symonds (Glenelg). Pritchard would play 211 games and share in the 1988, 1989 and 1991 premierships, but the other four managed just three games between them. Collingwood went for Grant Fielke (West Adelaide), David Robertson (North Adelaide), Craig Kelly (Norwood), Brendan Hogan (Assumption College) and Wayne Tanner (Norwood). Only Kelly, a 122-gamer and 1990 premiership team member, had a big impact, and ironically, he would end up managing my promotional affairs late in my career, when he was a key executive with Elite Sports Properties. It's a small world, football.

I needn't have worried about the draft — not that I did anyway. Before the draft I'd gone to work in my new job as a teller at the National Bank at Rosny. I'd met Arthur Wilson at a coffee shop near the bank and he'd given me an undertaking that Fitzroy would draft me if the opportunity arose. Arthur had shown most interest in me before the draft but if there had been the live media coverage the draft has today, and I'd been able to follow the selections, I might have been worried. For their first pick the Lions chose Jason Taylor (New Norfolk). They followed that with my clubmate Matty Armstrong. Then they switched to Adelaide to choose Chris Duthy (Glenelg). It wasn't until No. 50 — in a draft which would only go to 65 — that I got my chance. Immediately afterwards, though, the draft number was irrelevant. You were either a listed AFL player or you were not. Arthur rang me with the news that I was in, and I was happy. Fitzroy had finished third in 1986 after a good run of sustained success in the early 1980s. It was a good place to be heading.

But not just yet. After several long talks with Huddo, we decided I should play another season with Hobart before heading to Melbourne. It wasn't an issue for Matty

Armstrong. He was a much more accomplished player than me, and was already playing state football. He was ready to take the next step. But I felt I needed to get a few more kicks in Tassie before I took on the best in the country. So, with Fitzroy's blessing, I played in Hobart in 1987 with the express goal of earning a state jumper.

I did that, and it was a day I'll never forget. I was chosen to play against the VFA at Junction Oval in a side coached by Andy Bennett and captained by Greg Farquhar. We caught a 6.30am flight to Melbourne, but as we neared Tullamarine we were told that the airport was closed due to fog. We circled for two hours until, running low on fuel, we were diverted to Canberra. We landed there and had a healthy lunch of hot chips and sauce — they'd run out of everything else — before reboarding the flight for Melbourne. Tullamarine was still closed, but not for too much longer; eventually we were given a clearance to be the first plane to land. It was 2pm before we got to the ground. The game started an hour late, at 3pm. Not surprisingly, the VFA jumped us early and beat us by about the same margin as the early lead. I started on the wing, but when Ian Paton, a 155-game Hawthorn ruckman and dual premiership player, was injured in an early collision with 226-game ex-St Kilda giant Jeff Sarau I suddenly found myself playing in about the only position I'd never really played: ruck. I was thrown around a bit at the boundary throw-ins and I wasn't too keen on contact at the centre bounces, so I was happy to pick up a few touches around the ground and not get hammered by my giant opponent. It was great to have played my first state game.

So, after my second TFL season with Hobart — we finished fourth — I headed to Melbourne in November 1987. Fitzroy and the big time, here I come. I didn't know if I was really ready, and I didn't know what to expect. But I was excited. What for most of my life had been something I watched with keen interest from afar had suddenly become an infatuation. I wanted to play at the highest level. To do as my little mate Matty Armstrong had done. 'Dogsy' was already a 20-game veteran, and despite Fitzroy finishing 11th in the 14-team competition, he was loving every minute of it.

3

SIX YEARS AT FITZROY

They called Fitzroy 'the people's club'. And with very good reason. It didn't matter that we didn't have a lot of the comforts and luxuries of other clubs or that we seemed to have this ongoing battle for survival. It didn't matter that the support was not big in numbers. They were passionate and loyal. The players and the supporters made it a special club.

I had six fantastic years at Fitzroy, from 1988 to 1993. I played 120 of a possible 130 games. Only once did we threaten the finals. In 1989 we were fifth with three games to play, but we ended up sixth — one win plus percentage outside the top five. Overall, we finished 12th–6th–12th among 14 teams in my first three years; and

14th–10th–11th from 15 teams in my last three years. As silly as this might sound, it didn't really matter. Sure, you play to win. Sure, you're disappointed when you lose. Especially when you get thumped. But that didn't mean I didn't love the place. And all because of the people.

There is and always will be a very special bond among the Fitzroy players of my era. Twelve years after I left the club I still keep in regular contact with a lot of ex-teammates. They are mates you don't have to talk to every second day to remain close to, and yet I talk to a lot of them weekly. And I know that if ever I need a hand they wouldn't hesitate.

I got myself into trouble once because of a Fitzroy friendship. Roosy had played his 250th game in Round 3, 1994. Ironically, it was against Brisbane at Western Oval (later Whitten Oval). I should have been playing against him but was sidelined with a broken collarbone. Three weeks later, on 30 April, there was a tribute function for him at the Botanical Hotel at South Yarra in Melbourne. The Bears had played Adelaide at the Gabba that day and I had kicked five goals in an 11 point loss. I flew to Melbourne for the function. Paul had been a magnificent support to me and a great friend over a long, long time and I wasn't going to miss his occasion.

But on the following Monday, at the Bears review meeting, coach Robert Walls let me know that he didn't think it was the right thing to do. It went something like, 'You're a Brisbane player now — not a Fitzroy player — don't forget it.' Craig Starcevich had organised an informal dinner for a few of the players in Brisbane on the Saturday night and because of Roosy's tribute I hadn't been there. It wasn't a compulsory function, and wasn't attended by more than a handful of players. But Wallsy had a point to make. I thought he was wrong and immediately after the meeting I approached him and told him I disagreed. I could see where he was coming from and could understand it. Here was this recruit fraternising with the enemy: his old club. But my loyalties were 100 per cent to Brisbane, and whether I was playing for Brisbane, Melbourne, Adelaide or Wynyard I would have attended Roosy's tribute dinner.

The Fitzroy bond isn't a premiership bond, but it is similar. Why? I've been asked a lot of times and I don't really know. It's special in a different way. It's all to do with the people. They are real quality. Perhaps, too, it was because through the hard times we had to rely so much on each other. We didn't have a lot else to fall back on, so we had to find a way to try to compete with the better sides.

We established a premiership-type unity within the core group. We trained and played together, and away from football we socialised together. Always did and always will.

Fitzroy's supporters were just as special. We didn't have a lot of them, but what we lacked in quantity we more than made up for in quality.

Fitzroy hadn't won a premiership since 1944 and weren't like the glamour clubs Carlton, Collingwood and Essendon. Yet the loyalty and enthusiasm of their members had to be seen to be believed. Football wasn't just a part of their lives — it was their lives. Their mood going to work on a Monday morning depended on whether we'd won or lost. But they'd be back the following week, regardless of the weekend's results, cheering as if we were on a 10-game winning streak and good things for the finals again.

There was also one extra special person I met through my days at Fitzroy — my future wife, Peta Embling. Pete was a long-time friend of Ross Lyon's girlfriend at the time, Donna Le Page, and one night after a game against St Kilda at Princes Park Donna had invited Pete out to dinner. Ross asked me to come, too. It was 15 July 1989. I'll never forget it — and not because it was the start of a five-game winning streak, the longest I would enjoy at Fitzroy.

Rossy and I had a few beers at Lord Jim's Hotel, North Fitzroy, which was owned by teammates Scott Clayton and Matt Rendell. So we were a bit late — and a bit jovial. We were to meet the girls outside the movies, but by the time we got there the movie had started and they'd already gone in. 'We're looking for two girls who might have been waiting for us,' we told the usher, who knew exactly whom we were talking about. We stumbled in the dark but she took us straight to where they were sitting. After watching *Indiana Jones and the Temple of Doom*, the sequel to *Raiders of the Lost Ark*, we went to dinner at the Flower Drum in Chinatown, then next door to Harley's Bar for a few drinks, and finally to one of the nightclubs in King Street.

Before this, though, life for me at Fitzroy began with six weeks of living in Kings Way Motel, South Melbourne, as a guest of the club. I was a tall, skinny kid, weighing about 85kg, still wet behind the ears, happy just to be living my football dream.

Then I moved into a nice big house at East Brighton, just off the Nepean Highway, near the intersection of South Road. It had to be a big house because in it were Tassie boys Matty Armstrong, Michael and Brendon Gale and yours truly, plus South Australian recruit Darren

Kappler, and for a time Colac boy John Pekin, a brother of Fitzroy player Tim Pekin. Even former Royboy Jamie Cooper spent some time under the communal roof.

There were no girlfriends on the scene so we did everything together. And when we didn't visit the nearby Marine Hotel for a counter meal we'd share the cooking. And the chores. Even if big Benny Gale was a Richmond player among five Lions. Kapps was clearly the most domesticated of the group, but despite his best endeavours, the place occasionally resembled a pigsty. It really got under Kapps' skin. The rest of us managed to live with the mess. Just.

Shopping was always an issue. We'd go together and have a bit of fun until we had to pay the bill. With three trolleys full of food it was always plenty. We were very happy when Campbell's came on board as a club sponsor because the Player of the Week got a big carton of soup. At one stage, between us we won it five weeks in a row, so the pantry was full for a couple of months.

One of the odd things Fitzroy supplied its players with was undies. An added bonus, I guess, but it made life a bit difficult for us, because the entire household had the same white undies and it became a question of who could find a pair first.

I felt right at home at Fitzroy from the outset. Coach David Parkin was a welcoming type and he and Arthur Wilson always made sure we were OK. And besides, my mullet, very much the hairstyle rage back then, stacked up beautifully alongside those of Matt Rendell, the former captain, and Paul Roos, the current captain. I was with the strength.

I did have one problem — I'd lost my licence for six months. So in my early days in Melbourne I caught a lot of trains. I was lucky the public transport system was so good. And even luckier that I'd been able to arrange a transfer with the National Bank and was working nice and centrally on St Kilda Road, not far from where we trained at Lakeside Oval.

Gavin Hopper, in charge of the Fitzroy fitness program through the late 1980s, trained us very hard. It was a long, hard slog. I was just a kid so I did what I was told. And the more experienced Armstrong, Michael Gale and Kappler were ever generous with their advice. I loved the training, although not so much the mountain of running. Still, it was a great feeling driving home after a big session being part of the AFL. Some days we'd do one session before work and another session after work. There were no professional footballers in those days.

At least in the 1987–88 summer I managed not to cover myself in embarrassment, which was more than I could say for an incident 12 months earlier. It was my first training session with Fitzroy after Dogsy Armstrong and I had been drafted together from Hobart. While I was deciding whether to make the move to Victoria in 1987, we'd flown over to do some pre-Christmas training and we met the players on the Saturday morning at Lakeside Oval. They were to do a triathlon at nearby Kerford Road Beach. Because we didn't have bikes, we jogged 2km down to the starting point. We were feeling a bit uncomfortable, not really knowing too many people, but we started to mingle with the playing group warming up on the sand. As we looked around, we were a bit surprised to see Dale Weightman. And then Mark Lee and Jimmy Jess, among others. Oh no, I thought. We'd inadvertently joined the Richmond players, who by chance were doing exactly the same thing on the same beach at the same time. The Fitzroy boys were 400m further down the sand. We snuck sheepishly away. Never had a 400m jog been more embarrassing.

This was in the days before regimented training gear, so when I came back for my first full pre-season I was happy to accept a proper uniform. Shorts, socks, T-shirts, singlets, the lot. At least I wouldn't make that mistake again.

Initially I was allocated jumper No. 26. It had been worn by my former East Brighton housemate Jamie Cooper, who had played 26 games for Fitzroy from 1984 to 1987. He'd departed to begin a career that would ultimately make him the official artist of the AFL, responsible for the Team of the Century paintings for the League and most clubs. Jumper numbers didn't really worry me, but when Doug Barwick, who had worn No.11 at Fitzroy, switched to Collingwood over the summer I asked for and was given No. 11. I'd worn No. 11 in Hobart and thought I may as well stick with the same number.

At the Bicentennial Championships in Adelaide, held in March before the 1988 AFL season, I wore No. 10 because Barwick, a fellow Tasmanian, was in No. 11. That was a fantastic experience for a young fella still feeling his way. The Tassie side, coached by Robert Shaw, had a great mix of established players, including captain Rodney Eade, Michael Roach, 'Scratcher' Neal, Scott Clayton, my carnival roommate Ian Paton, and a bunch of kids like Darrin Pritchard, Matty Armstrong, Andy Lovell, Michael Gale, and Simon Minton-Connell who were just getting started.

My first State of Origin game for Tasmania against Northern Territory at Football Park on Wednesday,

2 March 1988, was a memorable one, but only because of an unusual and inadvertent incident. The coach had told me on Tuesday night at Norwood Oval that I'd trained my way into the side. I'd grabbed the last spot on the bench. So there I started, at 3.10pm, in front of next to nobody. We were the curtain-raiser to the Amateurs v ACT curtain-raiser. It was stinking hot and the sun was reflecting off the aluminium seats, which sat empty until the 8.10pm game between Victoria and Western Australia.

The NT side was captained by Maurice Rioli, with Michael McLean his deputy. It was full of talent and they had one thing in common. They could all run. The Territorians got off to a flyer, and the messages soon started coming from the coach's box down to the bench. Andy Bennett, a former Hawthorn and St Kilda player, was our assistant coach, and was filling in as runner. He spent a lot of time on the ground, and pretty quickly the inevitable happened: the phone rang when he was out in the middle. So, not knowing quite what to do but sitting closest to it, I answered it. 'Lynch,' I said. The coach paused for a moment before saying, 'Right, get Manson off and put Lynch to centre half forward.' So I jumped up off the bench, quickly got Bennett's attention and told him of Shawy's instruction. My first taste of Origin footy.

I learned later that, as I suspected, Robert Shaw had thought he was talking to Bennett when I introduced myself on the phone. And he'd thought Bennett was making a suggestion. But what was I to do? You have to make the most of every opportunity.

We got flogged by 11 goals, and then had to kick five goals to none in the final quarter to beat Queensland by 12 points two days later to avoid a wipe-out, but the carnival was a fantastic experience. It was the first time I'd seen at close quarters what AFL footballers were about. How big and strong they were, and how hard they worked. We had some fun, too, but it was an invaluable experience as a stepping stone to the AFL season that was to follow.

I signed my first contract with Fitzroy on 5 February 1988. I only know this because my father-in-law, Neil Embling, kept it. I'd planned to throw it out when I moved to Queensland — but he saved it and sent it up to me when I started on this book. It was a three-year deal, and in the first year I received a base salary of $5000 plus match payments of $600 (seniors), $150 (reserves) and $250 (official pre-season games). Plus four return airfares to Hobart. There were milestone payments of $1000 for five games and 10 games, and $2000 for 15 games. If I finished in the top six in the best and fairest I'd get an extra payment, ranging from $1000 for sixth up to $6000 for first. Plus I got $75 a week in board allowance, and a one-off signing fee of $5000.

The base salary increased to $6000 in 1989 and $7000 in 1990, senior match payments went up to $750 in 1989 and $900 in 1990, and the milestone payments increased slightly too. So I earned about $25,000 in year one, $23,000 in year two (no sign-on fee) and $32,000 in year three. Plus my weekly board. It was pretty good for a young bloke, although my bank wage was a bit of a bonus because I was known to grab an occasional sleep at lunch time.

In an early practice match for Fitzroy I just happened to play on the guy who, in his previous outing, had got the better of Hawthorn champion Dermott Brereton to win the Norm Smith Medal in the 1987 grand final. It was David Rhys-Jones. And he had a reputation for not showing a lot of consideration to raw 19-year-olds. I thought, what have I got myself into? Happily, I got a few kicks and my career didn't end before it had started.

My first official game for Fitzroy was in the reserves in Round 1, 1988. We played St Kilda at Princes Park, later known as Optus Oval, and I was late. I'd just got my licence back and had borrowed Michael Gale's trusty old

Kingswood. The rest of the household were playing in the seniors, so I left early by myself. But as I headed down the Nepean Highway I realised that I didn't really know where Princes Park was. Or how to get there. I got lost. After driving around for a while in a mad panic, I finally arrived, pulling into the carpark to find an anxious-looking Arthur Wilson. He didn't say much — just pointed me in the direction of the rooms. In I walked, and all of a sudden an eerie feeling hit me. There were a couple of trainers but nobody else. The team was already in the meeting room, being given their pre-game address from coach Garry Wilson. I knocked on the door sheepishly, apologised for being late, and didn't take in a word.

The coach, a Fitzroy legend, wasn't happy. In front of the entire group he told me I'd be starting on the bench. Not a good beginning, I thought. But after I quickly changed and explained what had happened, 'Flea' let me start on the ground. I kicked three goals and we won by 71 points. In Round 2 we lost by four points to Carlton at Princes Park. I kicked three goals and had a reasonable game, so I was in contention for senior selection.

I made my senior debut in Round 3 against Footscray at Western Oval. At least this time I didn't have to worry about finding the ground by myself. I could hitch a ride with the boys. I'd been at the club on the Tuesday night when David Parkin pulled me aside and told me I was in. I floated around the place for the next few hours; it was good to get the news from the coach first-hand. Parko was a bloke I had enormous respect for — not just as a coach, but also as a person. He was ultra professional, but he didn't just care about his players as footballers; he was genuinely concerned for our development as people.

Listening to him talk now about me in my early days is interesting. He describes me as a 'quiet, shy kid who was a pure athlete, with a good vertical jump'. It's a nice way of saying I was a quiet, shy kid who could jump but really had no idea about football. And I didn't. There are two types of teenagers who come into the system these days — the pure footballers who have lived the game from an early age, and the athletic types who may have come from a different sporting background and don't have the same natural understanding of the game. Some were lucky enough to have both but I was more in the latter category in the early days.

Parko had told me on the Friday night I'd be starting on the ground at half forward in my first game. This was a Parkin ritual. He'd ring every player at home the night before a game to explain his role the following day. And maybe just to make sure we were home. The East Brighton boys represented a cost saving for the coach because he got to speak to four of us for the price of one call. Armstrong, Gale, Kappler and Lynch. Once he even got mixed up. He thought he was speaking to Dogsy when in fact it was 'Butch' Gale. They didn't dare let on; they just carried on with the charade and exchanged instructions later.

Parko's other trademark was the reams of paperwork he did. He was a long way ahead of his time. While it became common practice from the late 1990s for players to get a full and detailed report on the opposition side each week, it was the exception in 1988.

On debut, I was picked up by Steve Wallis. I was 12cm taller than him but we weighed about the same. My first kick was a skier from general play towards the goal square. Nothing special. But my second was a goal. A drop kick goal. All thanks to Leon Harris. He'd won the ball and was running towards goal 30m out and could easily have had a shot, but looking after the new boy, he gave me a handpass. And for some inexplicable reason I got just inside the goal square and kicked a drop kick. How stupid would I have looked if I'd missed? Fortunately, I didn't. I finished with two goals in a 51-point loss — but for 16 years I'd convince myself it was four goals! Not a bad start,

I used to think. My illusions were shattered by research for this book. At least my career was up and going.

I played six in a row, including my first interstate trip to take on Brisbane at Carrara in Round 6 and my first win over Sydney at Princes Park in Round 7, when I had to bluff my way through our club song because I had no idea of the words. In Round 8 I felt the selectors' axe, but a week later I was back in the seniors, and there I stayed almost for the rest of the season. It was embarrassing, really, because I didn't deserve a spot. I'd shown a bit early and I've got no doubt the coach stuck with me as an investment in the future. Often, too, I'd get a lot more ground time than my form warranted.

John Ironmonger, a ruckman who had won the 1983 Sandover Medal playing with East Perth, had joined Fitzroy from Sydney in 1988. This meant trouble for Matt Rendell, an all-time great of the club. He'd won the best and fairest in 1982–83 and was captain in 1985–86–87, yet in '88 he played just one solitary game. Parko used to take a squad of 22 or 23 into the team meeting on the Thursday night, and announce the final side. And every week 'Bundy' would walk out shaking his head. He'd been fantastic to me when I first joined the club and I felt terrible that I was getting a game and he was missing out.

One day, late in the season, after Parko had delivered his almost weekly bad-news bulletin, Matty and I walked out of the room together. He looked at me, shook his head and said, 'You're a bloody genius.' I didn't feel like a genius. I'd been hoping he'd put me out of my misery and give me a run in the reserves, but that didn't come until Round 24, which was Parko's last game at the club. We'd finished 12th, but he'd done a great job for me and I couldn't have hoped for a better mentor to begin my career.

It got pretty cold in the middle of winter in Melbourne, even for a Tasmanian boy, and our big East Brighton home was freezing, with only a fireplace for warmth. It was no push-button electric job: you actually had to lay a fire. And that meant timber. For a while we bought some packets of wood from the service station up the road, but that got a bit expensive. So occasionally, when it was really cold, we burned the fence palings from behind the garage. And then Michael Gale used the Kingswood to knock over a decent-sized tree in the backyard. We didn't have an axe, so we broke off the small branches and fed the trunk into the fire bit by bit as it burned. When we'd exhausted the supply of fence palings and the tree we thought we'd have to go cold. But Dogsy Armstrong had other ideas. He went out the back, and all of a sudden we hear crash, bang, and back he comes with a few pieces of timber just right for the fire. It was the outdoor table and chairs that Mick Conlan had given me after I'd paid him $100 for an old bed when I moved into the house. I never had the heart to tell Mick. Sorry, mate. But at least it kept us warm for a few nights.

Mick Conlan was a legendary bloke. He played for ACT but he was actually born in Tasmania, so the clan of Armstrong, Gale, Kappler, Clayton and Lynch happily claimed him. He worked really hard in the gym, and when he finished he'd get back into his suit, put on his tie and do his hair before leaving. 'Going out, Mick?' we'd ask. 'No — just going home.' One of the most immaculately dressed footballers you'd meet.

Scotty Clayton taught me a few things in my first couple of years. One of them was about towels. More particularly, other players' towels. Scotty told me it was only the naive rookies who took their own towels to training. The veterans didn't trouble themselves with such niceties; they always managed to borrow someone else's towel. If only I'd learned this a bit earlier, it might have spared me all those nights where I'd get in from training and find a wet, screwed-up towel in the bottom of my bag.

In 1989 Rod 'Curly' Austin took over as Fitzroy coach. He was a 220-game Carlton premiership player who had been coaching Footscray reserves. I had immediate respect for him because once he'd kept the great Peter Hudson goal-less. He brought with him a new reserves coach: Robert Shaw, another Tasmanian, who had played 51 games at Essendon and was Tasmania's State of Origin coach. It was the beginning of what would be my most successful year at Fitzroy in a team sense, although things took a little while to fall into place.

In Round 2 against Collingwood at Princes Park I sat on the bench until time-on in the final quarter. It had gone beyond the stage where I was hoping to get a run. By then I just wanted to get out of there. But Gary Pert, the Victorian State of Origin fullback, was injured and Curly sent me on in his place. My first taste of life in the defensive goal square. I must have been a bit loose, though, because I still managed to kick a goal.

I got a full-scale introduction to fullback play the following week against St Kilda at Waverley. And what an introduction it was. I was playing at half forward and doing all right. I'd even kicked three goals, so I was pretty disappointed when five minutes into the third quarter I was dragged. Taken from the field. When I got to the bench I was told the coach wanted to talk to me and I was thinking something like, 'Good — I wouldn't mind having a chat to him, too.' Then he told me he wanted me to have a quick spell before I went to fullback. I was to play on Tony Lockett, who had already kicked eight goals on Perty, the best fullback in the country. Or 8.6, to be precise. I was dumbfounded. Me, a kid from Wynyard, who had played all of two minutes at fullback in his entire career after spending almost an entire game on the bench, going to play on 'Plugger'? Rod Austin was renowned for his lousy jokes, but this was ridiculous.

I was maybe 89kg by then, and during the two minutes I had to prepare, I made one wise decision. I couldn't possibly hope to match the big fella for strength. He was 100kg-plus and would have thrown me around like a rag doll. So I decided to play him from a few metres behind. I'd make sure he couldn't get hold of me in a wrestle and I'd back myself and my pace to catch him on the lead and get a fist in. Well, it worked. Lockett finished the day with 8.8. He let me off a couple of times when he missed, but he didn't add to his goal tally. He hardly said a word to me. I'd like to think it was because of his new-found respect, but he probably didn't even know who I was. And so began a long history of head-to-head meetings which I always enjoyed. Even if the big man was the leading goal-kicker of all time.

We got to Round 20, having won five in a row and needing to beat fifth-placed Collingwood to give ourselves a real chance of making the finals. More than 42,000 people, easily the biggest crowd I'd played in front of to that point, packed Waverley for what was a mini-final. We lost by 33 points, and worse still, Richard Osborne, Fitzroy's leading goal kicker for the fourth year in a row, did his knee. It was a shocking hyper-extension that would sideline him for almost 11 months. And as if that wasn't enough, we lost to lowly Brisbane the following week. Season over.

Happily, though, there were two highlights which came on the same day in September. The reserves won the 1989 premiership and I won the AFL Mark of the Year. It was announced on grand final day, although I didn't find out until I was enjoying a celebratory drink with the reserves at Lord Jim's Hotel.

The mark had come on a wet and muddy Sunday afternoon in Round 16 against North Melbourne at the MCG. It had been a good day all round, because I had kicked six goals. The conditions were diabolical — it makes me embarrassed when I think how much modern-day players complain if the surface isn't bowling-green perfect. This was like rolled mud. And that's being generous. Matt Rendell kicked the ball from the members' flank to about 40m from goal at the city end. I was playing on John Law in a forward pocket and had a chance to get a bit of a run at it. A fortuitous Law push meant I got a fair sit on a pack which included teammates Paul Roos and David Strooper, and North's Ben Buckley. Somehow I managed to time things just right and I took it on my chest, sitting on their shoulders. Even had a nice soft landing.

Most of the senior players gathered behind the goals to watch the reserves grand final. (This was the day Geelong played in the Under 19s preliminary final and the reserves and seniors grand final — and lost all three by a kick or less.) Fitzroy, coached by Robert Shaw, were down at half-time but came back from nowhere. It was the last game for stalwarts Mick Conlan, Leon Harris, Ross Thornton and Mark Scott, and prompted some serious celebrations. I reckon half the team bunked that week in the home at Mt Waverley which I'd bought in 1989 with Darren Kappler and Darren Louttit, a former Melbourne player who had crossed to Fitzroy in 1988. By then Louttit had left, Kapps had bought his share, and Carl Dilena — pick No. 3 in the 1988 national draft, from Sturt in Adelaide — was renting the spare room. He'd played in the reserves premiership side so there was plenty to celebrate.

But it all came to a shuddering halt three days later. On Tuesday, 3 October 1989 I was awoken by a call from Dad, with the news that Fitzroy and Footscray were to merge and become the Fitzroy Bulldogs. He'd heard it on the radio.

It was a bombshell. There had been a bit of talk but nothing formal, at least not down among the second-year players like me. We'd even played Footscray in the last round and nothing had been said. All of a sudden the place was as flat as could be. We were shattered. We were a bunch of young kids, still finding our feet in League football, and we were devastated by the news that we were about to be split up. What that would have meant for me, I have no idea. I never heard anything, so I assumed I wasn't to be part of the merger plans. Where I was going to finish up was anyone's guess.

In researching this book I learned via Max Kelleher, Fitzroy chief executive at the time, that in fact negotiations had been going on for several months. Only two people from each club, plus a small and still secret delegation at the AFL, were aware of it, and they were sworn to secrecy. They didn't even tell their wives, according to Max.

The deal was done. The Fitzroy Bulldogs were to wear what was essentially the Fitzroy jumper, with a yellow band around the middle in the style of the old Footscray jumper. Today a sample of the would-be jumper sits in the MCC Museum.

According to Max, the merged club was to be based at Western Oval and would continue to operate the recruiting zones of Fitzroy and Footscray. The debt of both clubs was to be wiped and there would be sufficient capital to alleviate the financial pressure both clubs were feeling. The team, to be coached by Fitzroy coach Rod Austin, would have comprised the cream of the two playing lists. It would have been a powerful side. I was even going to get a contract, apparently.

Max, Fitzroy CEO from 1988–91, told me he was to have been the CEO of the new club had it not fallen over when the cone of silence was broken the night before the announcement was due. Apparently Footscray chief executive Denis Galimberti got wind of it and next thing it was in the media. That, he told me, denied the merger insiders the opportunity to present the story properly and to sell it to the relevant parties. Each of the four insiders had a list of people they were to contact the night before the announcement but before this could be done properly it was out.

There was a massive public uproar, with AFL chief executive Ross Oakley bearing much of the brunt of it. There were even 'Up Yours Oakley' and 'Merge Oakley Into Outer Space' bumper stickers, and, as I learned later, Oakley had a bloke who was stalking him outside his home. Not a pleasant business but indicative of the passion that went with League football.

A lobby group at Footscray took the matter to court and the court ruled that the agreement was invalid. This bought enough time for the Footscray supporters to rally around and raise enough money to save their club. And 21 days after the League had announced the merger they were forced to do a back-flip and confirm that both clubs would carry on as separate entities in 1990.

Fitzroy emerged from the would-be Footscray merger in much the same shape we'd always been in: struggling for money but full of hope and spirit. I played every game in the season for the first time in 1990. We finished 12th, and the only real highlight came in the State of Origin game against Victoria at North Hobart Oval.

The year before, 1989, Tasmania, coached by Roland Crosby and captained by Scott Wade, had led Victoria at half-time. A fairytale win was on the cards until Hawthorn game-breaker Gary Ayres went into the centre and cut us apart. They steamrolled us by 57 points, with Paul Salmon kicking seven goals and Ayres, the Victorian captain, kicking four. The visitors got off North Hobart Oval before any of us young whipper-snappers, who had grown up idolising the Big V, could suggest trading jumpers. I did get one from Gary Pert, but only after the game. He had plenty anyway.

In 1990, back at North Hobart, the Tassie boys were a year older and a year wiser. And a year stronger. Now coached by Robert Shaw, and with Hawthorn's Darrin Pritchard at the helm, we led at half-time again, but this time we weren't about to be overrun. The ground was full and the atmosphere was sensational. The fans went crazy, chanting 'Tassie, Tassie' as we got home by 33 points. It was only the second time Tasmania had beaten Victoria, and the first since 1961. I'd played at fullback on North Melbourne's John Longmire; Victorian coach David Parkin gave me his best player award. One for old times' sake. I must have enjoyed myself, too, because I was the last player off the ground. I stayed out there chatting with friends and family, and by the time I forced my way down the packed players' race I'd missed the coach's post-game address. There was no jumper-trading this year either. Nobody wanted to give up this state jumper.

By the end of the 1990 season I'd played 58 AFL games, and felt that I belonged in League football. I'd learned a few things along the way. Two of the lessons were never to take anything for granted, and always to expect the unexpected. Like when Fitzroy tried to sell Paul Roos to Collingwood. I couldn't believe it. An icon of the game, one of the all-time Fitzroy greats, and they were prepared to off-load him to the enemy! I guess it said something about the perilous state of the club's finances.

Roosy, at the time dating an American girl named Tami, later to become his wife, was enjoying his annual end-of-season holiday in the United States when he received a call from his manager, Damien Smith. He'd been given two options by Fitzroy: take a 33 per cent pay cut or be traded to the club of his choice. The third option was to try his luck in the pre-season draft. He wasn't going to take such a big pay cut, and Damien told him that Collingwood had already expressed a strong interest, so they agreed to pursue that option. Roosy decided it was best to be in Australia while everything was happening so he flew home.

But it wasn't quite as easy as it might have been, because the Magpies were unable to work a deal with Fitzroy. No

Collingwood players were prepared to be part of the trade that would get Roosy to Victoria Park. Ron McKeown had been earmarked as a possible target but it didn't happen. It all fell through. So, having not heard personally from anyone at Fitzroy throughout the whole deal, Roosy rang the club. He wanted to know where he stood. They told him he was a Fitzroy player. What about his contract? The club was prepared to continue his existing deal.

So he flew back to the United States and sent them a fax resigning as captain. If they didn't really want him as a player, he didn't feel comfortable being captain, he told them. But he'd be back for training in January. Not a good situation. But it wasn't the only such incident.

Gary Pert had suffered his second serious knee injury in the last game of season 1990 and he, too, felt the sting of the financial pressure. Facing 12 months out of the game in what was scheduled to be his life membership year, he was told by the club that even though he was under contract, he wasn't going to be paid.

Perty was a favourite son of Fitzroy. An All-Australian, 1989 best and fairest winner and vice-captain. A genuine superstar. And we didn't have too many of them. He'd played 163 games with the Lions after making his debut as a 16-year-old in 1982. Eight times he'd worn the Big V of

Victoria. And his father Brian had played 125 games for the club from 1954 to 1965 and was a life member.

He was devastated, rightly. They didn't even try to broker a deal to ease the financial pressure. It was just this heavy-handed edict. When the Roos trade fell over, they offered Pert instead. Finally, the club admitted that the original contract was valid and tried to make peace with him, even to the point of asking him to go back and play. But the damage was done. He couldn't go back. And at the end of 1991 he was traded to Collingwood for selections No. 2 and No. 25 in the national draft. He went on to become a valuable 70-game player with the Magpies over four years from 1992.

Robert Shaw took over as senior coach in 1991 and immediately made changes. Roosy, after three years as captain, was replaced by Richard Osborne. A new-look understudy leadership group included Ross Lyon, John Blakey and me.

Shawy was a tremendously astute coach. He was a great football thinker, and tactically he was as smart as any. Personally, I had a huge wrap on him. I'd enjoyed my time under him with the Tasmanian State of Origin side, I got along with him well, and I relished the encouragement he gave me to play a variety of roles in any game.

But it was a long, hard year. Three times we lost by more than 100 points — to Melbourne in our first game, Round 2 (131 points — we had a bye in Round 1), to Hawthorn in Round 6 (157 points) and to Hawthorn again in Round 21 (126 points). And there was also a 99-point loss to West Coast in Round 9.

The first loss to Hawthorn was Fitzroy's biggest-ever defeat. It came in our first game at North Hobart Oval — the club had initiated a campaign to develop a supporter base in Tasmania. Playing at fullback, I got a stiff neck as I watched 36 goals go over my head.

Darren Jarman and Ben Allan kicked seven goals apiece for Hawthorn, and Jason Dunstall, my opponent all day, bagged six. A long day for the defenders.

We went back to North Hobart in Round 13 to play St Kilda. This time I was confronted by Tony Lockett. I felt I kept a close check on him all day. I spoiled well and won a fair bit of the footy. He had eight kicks and kicked eight goals, and the Saints won by 13 points. So, for two visits home to Hobart I'd had two games in which I thought I'd done all right and had still conceded 14 goals. And the team had conceded 53.

Our second visit to Tasmania was memorable for more than just Lockett's unerring conversions. It was probably the only time in modern football that a travelling team stayed with local residents.

I'm not kidding. The club said it was trying to get the Tasmanian people to embrace Fitzroy, but I'm not so sure. Anyway, when we arrived at Hobart Airport, the names were read out and off went the players to their homes for the next couple of days. I hadn't experienced anything like this since I visited Melbourne with the North Tasmanian Under 12 soccer team and stayed with a family at Mulgrave. Happily, being a local, I'd arranged to stay with my stepbrother Steven Wright, and I had the house to myself as he went off to work. But we heard some nightmare stories of younger players without the confidence to speak up being taken on a sightseeing visit to the top of Mt Wellington on the way to the game. Jimmy Wynd, renowned for having to visit the bathroom during the night, was shattered to learn that at his billet's house it was a 15m walk across ice-covered grass to the outhouse. Not the average preparation for an AFL game, but it was that sort of year.

We'd got to Round 10 in dreadful shape. It was 0–9 Fitzroy against 9–0 Geelong. And yet we won by 21 points. The following week, playing Adelaide at Football Park, we felt we were robbed by the umpires. And I don't

think I'd say that about any other game I played. Three
diabolical free kicks inside the last four minutes not
only earned both men in white a stint in the reserves
the following week but also saw Rod Jameson kick
the winning goal for the Crows after the siren. So
incensed were the Fitzroy faithful that they spraypainted
AFL House with all sorts of obscenities. The old
Victoria–South Australia rivalry was also alive and well in
the Crows' first year in the national competition, and in
the intimidating Footy Park crowds likewise.

That was the thing about Fitzroy. We'd struggle against
the lesser sides but we travelled well interstate, especially
to Adelaide and Perth, and occasionally we'd manage to
pull off a giant upset. As in Round 24 against minor
premiers West Coast. Carrying the hopes of Victoria
against the emerging powerhouse from the west at Princes
Park, we won by 10 points to leapfrog Brisbane and avoid
the wooden spoon.

Most footballers in Melbourne through the late 1980s and
the early 1990s maintained a full-time job outside football.
I'd kept the bank job I'd transferred with from Hobart
until 1990, but by then I'd reached a stage where, while
not exactly threatening the chief executive's position, I

had enough responsibility to mean I struggled to get away in time for 5pm training each day.

So I looked around. Darren Kappler got a call from Stewey Duncan, an old mate, offering him a job in a new mobile phone business but Kapps already had a good job so he passed it on. In a few days I went from counting money to selling phones for the Cellular Service Centre on City Road, South Melbourne. The hours were more flexible, and I stayed there for 18 months. I worked alongside an ex-Telecom employee named David Costanzo, who headed the service department, and when Cellular Service Centre closed down, David and I went into the game ourselves. In 1990 we opened our own business, Greensborough Communications. It was based on Main Street, Greensborough, about halfway between where I lived (Eltham) and where David lived (Bundoora).

Though I can hear the chuckling, we did all right. This was when mobile phones were the new thing. It wasn't the hardest thing to sell them, and we pulled a wage each week. We quickly realised that we didn't need a shopfront — we did most business onsite — so we moved base to David's home. We operated there even after I moved into an apartment with Peta at Eltham. It was a good decision, because it freed up a lot of time to ride the go-karts at nearby South Morang. Even after I left Melbourne at the end of 1993, David kept the business running for several years, and he's still in the phone game today. I'm just not too sure what happened to the old company go-kart.

I'd never played in a senior final of any description, let alone a grand final, until the 1992 Foster's Cup pre-season night grand final. It was an experience in itself, and a fair effort for a side which had only won four games through the entire 1991 season. We won three on the trot to earn a crack at Hawthorn, the defending day and night premiers, at Waverley.

The Fitzroy supporters went crazy. It was a chance for the club to earn some silverware. We had the majority of the support in the second-biggest crowd ever for a night grand final, but sadly, we finished on the wrong end of a 19.14 (128) to 8.15 (63) scoreline. In reality, the game was much closer than that. A 10-minute surge late in the second quarter and a similar burst in the second half made the difference, as a star-studded Hawk forward line — which included Jason Dunstall, Dermott Brereton, Tony Hall and Darren Jarman — proved too good. My old Hobart mate Paul Hudson won the Michael Tuck Medal as best on ground, and I was left to wait nine years to play in any sort of premiership decider again. It was a lesson: play for the moment, because you never know when or if the moment will come around again.

Season 1993 was my best at Fitzroy. Alternating from one end of the ground to the other, I kicked 68 goals and was chosen in the All-Australian team at fullback. And I won the best and fairest, after having finished sixth, second and equal third in the previous three years. I was favourite for the Brownlow Medal on the day of the count, but though I started to wonder as the odds kept shortening, deep down I knew I was never a chance. Something to do with a terrible habit of arguing with the umpires. I got 10 votes and finished a tie for 22nd — as close as I'd ever get.

It was the year Jason Dunstall, Gary Ablett and Tony Modra all kicked 100 goals — the first time three players had topped the ton in the same season since Huddo, Peter McKenna and Alex Jesaulenko did it in 1970. Modra got 129, Ablett 124 and Dunstall 123. With Peter Sumich, John Longmire and Sav Rocca all getting 70-plus, and Tony Lockett getting 53 in 10 games, it wasn't a good year for fullbacks.

Still, I really enjoyed playing on the superstar goal-kickers. There is no better challenge than testing yourself against the best, and this was an era of freakish quality. Toss in guys like Stephen Kernahan and at centre half forward Wayne Carey and the time was right to move to the other end of the ground.

As season 1993 closed I had no idea it would be my last at Fitzroy. It was almost as if someone was giving me a fantastic send-off: we won our last four games — a winning streak we'd only bettered once during my time (when we won five on the trot in 1989).

In Round 19 we beat eventual preliminary finalists Adelaide at Princes Park, followed by wooden-spooners Sydney at the SCG, 13th-placed Brisbane at Princes Park by 104 points — my only triple-figure win for Fitzroy — and finally 10th-placed Melbourne at the MCG. And all that after I'd kicked a career-best eight goals against Footscray the week before.

I walked off the MCG on the afternoon of Sunday, 29 August 1993, for what would be the last time as a Fitzroy player, a pretty happy fella. I was a 120-game player who was loving life as an AFL footballer. But I knew I had a massive decision to make.

4

THE MOVE TO BRISBANE

Leaving Fitzroy was just about the hardest thing I've done. I loved the club, I loved the people and I loved the fans. They were real, and for six years it was home. As much as you play football to win, it wasn't the end of the world that we hadn't been overly successful, because we were in it together.

I'd had plenty of opportunities to leave in the early 1990s. Footscray, Richmond and St Kilda had made the strongest approaches. The Bulldogs were very active in recruiting, and they had a big crack at me after the failed Fitzroy–Footscray merger of 1989. They offered really good money. At St Kilda I met with coach Ken Sheldon and my long-time mentor Peter Hudson, who was football manager there at the time. And at Richmond I met with general manager Cameron Schwab shortly after I'd installed a mobile phone into his car and the cars of several Tiger colleagues.

I listened to the offers but didn't think seriously about going. For me, none of it was ever about money; all I cared about was knowing for sure that I was going to get what I was contracted to get. Call me naive, but I never tried to negotiate an increase on what the club offered. I did my own contract, without a manager, and considered myself fortunate to be paid good money to play football. After all, what sports-crazy bloke in his early 20s wouldn't love living in Melbourne and playing footy with the terrific bunch of guys we had at Fitzroy?

But over the years our 'family' started to disintegrate. One by one, good players left. Mick Conlan, Leon Harris and Ross Thornton retired at the end of 1989, and Scott Clayton followed in 1990. The club was struggling to make ends meet, but when they'd tried to trade Paul Roos and then Gary Pert to Collingwood they lost me a bit. It seemed unbelievable that two of the club's absolute greats were being offered for trade.

The exodus didn't stop there. Matt Rendell retired before being lured into a comeback by the Brisbane Bears,

Darren Kappler went to Sydney and even Tony Woods and Jason Taylor, largely untried at Fitzroy, were traded away. They later became good players, at Hawthorn.

At the end of 1992 John Blakey was traded to North Melbourne, and several months later Richard Osborne, a former Fitzroy captain and five-times leading goal-kicker, quit and joined Sydney. It was a never-ending slide that continued long after I'd left. Paul Broderick, Michael Gale and Jamie Elliott were off-loaded to Richmond in 1994, about the same time I moved on, and in 1995 Roosy went to Sydney, Ross Lyon joined me in Brisbane and Matty Armstrong went to North Melbourne. A mighty team it would have been if ever we could have reunited all the ex-Lions.

In those days players were paid once a year — on 1 December. We lived through the season on outside earnings. Most blokes had a job, although for some it was a bit tough and they looked forward to pay day. In my six years at Fitzroy, I was paid every cent due to me. Not always on time, but always paid.

But late in the 1993 season, president Dyson Hore-Lacy came to the players and told us that he couldn't categorically guarantee we'd be paid. The club's financial situation was worsening, and he'd been to the AFL and asked them to guarantee the players' payments. They wouldn't do it. Apparently under the AFL Commission guidelines they were not permitted to make this sort of financial commitment. Hore-Lacy said he'd do everything he could to make sure we were paid. He said he'd even tie himself to a light pole at the MCG if it looked as if the money wouldn't be available. I believed him, because he was as passionate as they came. He worked tirelessly, and certainly had the club's best interests at heart. You could never doubt his motivation or commitment.

The last straw for me at Fitzroy was the club's decision to play its home games at Footscray's Western Oval in 1994. It wasn't that the club was going to Western Oval. It was that we were leaving Princes Park. I'd played exactly half my 120 AFL games for Fitzroy at Carlton and loved it. Most importantly, we had a genuine home-ground advantage there. And now we were about to throw it all away.

It was a financial decision: apparently it was going to be cheaper for the club to play at Footscray. But that didn't sit well with me. We didn't have a lot of things going for us — surely we should hang on to something as tangible as our home ground.

One club which was finally starting to establish a genuine home-ground advantage was the Brisbane Bears.

They'd moved from Carrara on the Gold Coast to the Gabba in Brisbane in 1993, and while it was going to take some time, I could see that they were a club on the improve.

I'd taken a little more notice of them late in the season, after a game of golf with my old mate Scott Clayton, a fellow Tasmanian who had played 160 games with Fitzroy over 10 years and won the best and fairest before retiring in 1990. He was now working with the Bears as the club's Victorian manager, in charge of recruiting and Melbourne operations, and would shortly move to Brisbane to become director of football and assistant coach.

Scotty took Paul Roos and me out to Spring Valley Golf Club, a nice course out on the sand belt about 30 minutes southeast of Melbourne. He says he let me beat him by 10 shots just to make sure I was feeling good. Whatever makes him happy!

During the game he just happened to drop on me the possibility of going to Brisbane. The Bears and the Sydney Swans had been given, among other recruiting concessions, the right to recruit one uncontracted player before the 1994 pre-season draft. Essentially, this meant they could hand-pick an out-of-contract player — a rare treat in the modern era and its draft system.

It was a bombshell, but it came at an opportune time. I was terribly disappointed about the seemingly endless departure of close friends and good players from Fitzroy, as well as the pending move to Western Oval. Scotty's suggestion prompted me to sit down and really consider my options.

If I was going to make a change, my last choice would have been interstate. I loved Melbourne, and it was where my friends were. If I was going anywhere, I would have much preferred to join another Melbourne club. But that was out of the question. It was Brisbane and Sydney who had the draft concessions. So if I was going anywhere, it was north.

I had a brief chat with Swans general manager Ron Joseph. He flew to Melbourne to see me but it never went any further. As a boy from Wynyard, I'd found Melbourne a big change — I wasn't ready to live in Sydney. It was much too big. Too cosmopolitan.

But the Bears had real appeal. I'd spoken several times to Scott Clayton over the last few weeks of the season and had made the first of what would be a long and difficult sequence of decisions. I'd made up my mind that if things were right, yes, I was prepared to leave Fitzroy. So I accepted an obligation-free invitation to fly to Brisbane for a look around.

The fact that Scotty was an ex-teammate was a bonus. It gave me a starting point which I wouldn't have had with someone I didn't know. He was originally from the same club as me — Hobart Football Club — and I'd played alongside him at Fitzroy for three years. He used to own a pub in Melbourne with Matt Rendell, and while they didn't give too many beers away they did serve a good feed, and a few of the Fitzroy boys spent a bit of time there.

I'd played at the Gabba with Fitzroy in 1991 when it was a pear-shaped field surrounded by a greyhound track, and again in 1993, when it was just starting to take shape. By 1993 the visitors' rooms were good by AFL standards, but I'd never inspected the set-up which the Bears had for themselves under the old Social Club. Compared to most of the competition, it was sensational. I would never have contemplated joining the Bears if they'd still been at Carrara. Everything there was artificial and temporary, but the facilities at the Gabba were better than any I'd seen.

I had a good long chat with coach Robert Walls in his office. That was important, too, because it was always going to be a key factor in my decision. We had plenty to talk about. He was a former Fitzroy player and coach so we had some common ground. I was impressed. I liked the direction the club was taking: it was all about the future.

They were planning to build a side around the best young players they could get, topped off with a couple of established players. We talked about the role I might play, and what his immediate and medium-term aspirations were. It was exciting.

We went upstairs for a look at the Social Club, and who do I bump into but Brendan McCormack. Or Billy, as I used to call my ex-Fitzroy teammate, who was now playing with the Bears. 'What are you doing up here?' he asked. 'Just having a look around, Billy. Keep it to yourself.' It was all still confidential at this stage. We hadn't even discussed terms or conditions.

Billy told me he loved Brisbane, and that the Bears were on the rise. A young Victorian called Nathan Chapman had got plenty of good press during his first season, and there were some good wraps on a young redhead named Justin Leppitsch, who had done his knee early in the season. But Billy told me there was one better from Queensland. Michael Voss. He was going to be a superstar, Billy said.

I flew back to Melbourne thoroughly impressed. The facilities were great and the club was on the right track. They seemed to have an infrastructure that would allow them to be successful, and I knew the AFL, desperate to see football kick on in the northern states, was going to offer them every support. I felt comfortable with the key personnel. Scott Clayton I knew well anyway, but Robert Walls and CEO Andrew Ireland struck me as genuine and sincere football people. I had something to think about. But nothing had prepared me for the next stage of our talks.

I told Clayton over the phone a few days later I was willing to seriously consider a move to Brisbane, so he and Ireland put an offer together and flew to Melbourne. Well, you could have knocked me over with a feather. It was a 10-year football deal worth $1.8 million guaranteed — no secret because it was in the media at the time. There was a $150,000 base payment, and $1500 a game. Plus a $35,000 marketing job with Coca-Cola and help finding a job (in the travel industry) for Peta that was comparable to what she had in Melbourne at the time. And when I'd finished playing, the club would maintain my salary at the same level for the duration of the contract. Unbelievable.

Here I was, 25 years old, in the prime of my career, and they were offering me not just a chance to play with a club which I was confident would be successful, but the security that would allow me to set myself up for life. I was astonished.

The intention was that I'd play six or seven years with the Bears and then take an off-field role with the club, either in football or the marketing department, to complete the 10-year term. This was to help with the transition to life after football. I couldn't have asked for more. I'd earned good money at Fitzroy in 1993 — about $100,000 — but this was another level. I would be among the highest-paid players in the competition.

I'd taken on Damien Smith, Paul Roos' long-term manager, to give me a bit of guidance. Really, he was just there to help tie all the loose ends together. He'd met with Ireland and Clayton in a coffee shop in Lonsdale Street in the city before relaying the details of the offer to me. We went back to them together the following day. There was never any suggestion of trying to negotiate the terms of the contract. I was more than satisfied.

What I didn't realise at the time was that the Bears had offered a similar deal to Hawthorn's Jason Dunstall. They wanted the Queensland-born superstar to go home and finish his career with the Bears before joining the off-field team. But he was 29, and decided the timing wasn't quite right. It was a massive bonus for me.

By now it was all public. Somehow, it had leaked into the media. It never ceases to amaze me how that happens, but I'd quickly learned that secrets in football don't stay secret for too long. So the pressure started to mount. I'd never been one to make big decisions quickly or easily. And this was about as big as it would ever get.

I bounced it off a few people. Among them, there was Peter Hudson, by now at Hawthorn, and Mick Conlan, now a senior executive at Nike. I talked to them not because I thought they'd have anything extraordinary to add, but because they were people whose opinion I valued. I found it helped talking about it. Paul Roos, too. That was tough, because Roosy was Fitzroy captain, having been reinstated in 1992. While he insisted I shouldn't go, he did admit that it was a fantastic offer. My family just wanted what was best for me. And then there was Peta. It wasn't just my decision. It was our decision. We spent hours discussing it, and were really torn between life in Melbourne and the opportunities that had presented themselves in Brisbane.

Our life in Melbourne revolved heavily around the football club. After a game at Princes Park, when the younger guys would go out on the town, we'd go for a coffee or a gelato in Lygon Street with Paul and Tami Roos, Paul and Sharlene Broderick, John and Kelly Blakey or Duane and Janine Rowe. Just as the players had a special bond, the girls, too, were very close.

We'd been on holidays to Noosa with the Blakeys and once went sailing with Ross Lyon and his then girlfriend Donna in the Whitsundays. That was a story in itself. It only gets a run because everyone has to have a fishing story.

It was October 1990. Rossy, Donna, Peta and I had hired a 45-foot yacht called *Sam Jones* at Shute Harbour for 10 days and were planning a relaxation and fishing extravaganza. We had various catering options, from the 'all-inclusive' to the 'catch your own', but we backed ourselves to catch plenty so we only stocked up on the bare essentials. The Whitsundays are full of fish, we figured. We'd only be wasting our money if we bought meat.

I'd done a bit of sailing in Tasmania with my brothers and actually knew the difference between port and starboard, so with Rossy a more than capable first mate, we breezed through the obligatory sailing test with the instructor, just to prove to him that we were competent and his expensive yacht would be safe. I took us out nice and slowly, Rossy set the sails beautifully, around the buoy we went, back in. Perfect.

So the instructor hopped back into his little tinnie and off we went. Well, things didn't go quite so smoothly the second time. We got the mainsail up all right, but in a flash the headsail, which is meant to be fed out nice and slowly, unravelled itself full tilt. Someone must have let the rope go — it wasn't me, because I was at the wheel. Next thing we know it's full of wind, dragging us along out of control, and at the same time pulling us over into the water. On one side we had the sails almost getting wet, and on the other side we could see the keel just below the water line. We tried to wind in the headsail, but because it had run out at such a pace it had come off the spool. And as we tried to point her into the wind to stop we almost hit an island. Not good.

Luckily, the instructor hadn't gone too far. He saw our predicament and rescued us. 'I think it might be a good idea if you spend the first night in the harbour,' he said to us, his confidence down just a touch. So there we were, on the first night of our Great Barrier Reef excursion, tied up at a buoy 50m off the shore. It could only get worse if the toilets got blocked. They did. And if Rossy, when he took the girls to the mainland to shower the following morning, moored our tinnie in the spot reserved for a big catamaran from Hamilton Island. And if he almost knocked himself out as he ran back to move it after a couple of loud toots from the captain of the catamaran, slipping and smashing his head on the dinghy. He did.

But, committed sailors that we were, we managed to exit the harbour safely and find a beautiful, quiet little bay to anchor in that afternoon. We'd seen huge schools of tuna and were keen to get amongst them, so Rossy and I jumped into the dinghy and headed off to catch dinner. The lines hardly had time to get wet when bang, one went off. The rod was bent over. It was a big one. We pulled it in, wondering what it might be and fantasising about a feast. A turtle.

We got not another bite. Not then, and not for the next two days.

Four days into our holiday we had a problem with the water supply and had to make for Hamilton Island for fresh supplies. Not our fault this time, thankfully.

Just as we tied the yacht up in the Hamilton Island marina, who do we see but the Melbourne football trio of Garry Lyon, Brett Lovett and Rod Grinter. They'd taken the all-inclusive option on a big cruiser. They even had a captain to do the sailing. The first thing they said to us? 'How good is the fishing!' 'Great holiday,' we replied, not wanting to admit that we hadn't caught a thing.

This couldn't go on. Rossy and I headed straight to the bait shop. 'We're here on holidays and we've got to catch some fish,' we told the guy at the counter. 'What can we do?' He had just the plan — after selling us all the right hooks, bait and anything else fishing gurus might possibly need. 'Have you got a tinnie?' he asked. 'Yes? Right, moor it about 50m off the end of the airport runway at about 4pm and you'll be sweet.'

He was right. As soon as our lines hit the water we started getting some bites. No actual fish, but plenty of bites. And then we noticed something that was hard to miss. Making its way slowly down the runway towards us was a big Qantas jet. It was barely 100m from us when it turned around. The captain hit the throttle and all of a sudden it was as if we were in a washing machine. A hot washing machine. Water was splashing everywhere and the heat was stifling. As they do, the jet sat there for what seemed an eternity before it moved off down the runway and took off.

Rossy and I looked at each other, hardly saying a word. At least not any I can repeat. We pulled the lines in and headed back to shore. If we had a pair of binoculars we probably would have spotted the bloke from the bait shop and a few mates, Crown Lagers in hand, laughing their heads off.

We sheepishly had to tell the girls how we hadn't caught a thing (again). At least we were in port this time, so we could stock up on a few supplies. Just in case our luck didn't change. (It wasn't until 10 days later, when I went to get a haircut in Sydney, that I realised just how hot it had been in the jet's exhaust stream. The girl cutting my hair asked if I was a boilermaker. 'No, why?' I replied. 'It's just that your hair and eyebrows are all singed at the front.')

Six days to go on our fishing expedition. Things had to change. We were persistent, because the prospect of becoming vegetarians didn't exactly excite us. Every morning at eight o'clock and every afternoon at four o'clock Rossy and I would jump in the tinnie and head off to catch some fish. Nothing. Except for one spotted mackerel which we skull-dragged so far that by the time we got it in the boat it was dead.

Still, we had a lot of fun sailing around the Whitsundays until late in our holiday we came upon White Haven Beach. What a beautiful spot. Perfect white sand as far as the eye could see in either direction. And only two boats. Ours and another yacht on which a guy was setting up a wind-surfer. We trawled for fish for 45 minutes. Nothing. Again. And then, as the guy on the windsurfer sailed between us and his yacht, a reel went off. It bent right over and the line speared out at a rate of knots. Rossy and I looked at each other.

Again. As if to say, it couldn't happen, could it? But it had. We'd caught the wind-surfer. Eventually, the line broke and we headed back to the girls empty-handed. Again. And there was not another fish for the entire holiday.

So it wasn't just a football decision we were about to make three years later when we contemplated a move to Brisbane. It was a lifestyle decision. And our friends in Melbourne were people with whom we'd shared a lifetime of experiences in only six years.

Peta had been nothing but totally supportive, and would happily do whatever we considered was best for my football. But I didn't want to drag her to Brisbane knowing she wasn't totally happy and totally committed. We were living together at Eltham at the time and in May 1993 had made a long-term commitment by buying a house at East Hawthorn (which in fact we never lived in). We were in this together. We had to get it right.

At one stage Damien Smith asked to see a copy of Fitzroy's business plan and financial projections. Everything looked in order, but there were doubts about whether or not the club could achieve their projected results. After all, they had reported debts of $1 million after a 1992 trading loss of $350,000, and only a decision by Westpac to provide a $1.5 million guarantee had got the club into 1993.

Dyson Hore-Lacy had put a lot of pressure on me, saying publicly that if I left it would be the end of Fitzroy. But this was about my future and my family's future. If everything had been in order at Fitzroy, if they hadn't had ongoing money problems and ground problems, I would never have considered a move. But they did. So we decided to put the heat back on them. Damien asked the Fitzroy directors to personally guarantee the contract they had offered me. It was no more than they were asking me to do: back the club's ability to meet my contract. If they were so sure the club would achieve the financial results they had forecast, it wouldn't be a problem. They refused.

It got to mid-October and we still couldn't decide. We took a holiday at Noosa with John and Kelly Blakey. Suffice it to say that my dilemma dominated the conversation. The longer the to-ing and fro-ing went, the more frustrated I became. After dinner one night we got out a piece of paper and a pen and wrote down the pros and cons. It was a one-sided argument. Brisbane it was. We immediately felt a giant relief. Finally, a decision had been made.

I rang Peter Hudson to discuss it one last time the following day, and then phoned Damien Smith and asked him to advise Fitzroy. It was 19 October 1993. I was going to Brisbane.

There were still eight days until the end of the official AFL trade period. All of a sudden Fitzroy's position changed. Having originally said they would never trade me, now they offered to trade me to Essendon or Carlton. If they'd said this at the outset, everything would have been different. I would never have considered Brisbane. But by now I felt I was too far down the track with the Bears. It would have been wrong to renege on my commitment. We had a deal, and if that meant I had to wait until the pre-season draft, when the Bears could claim me as an out-of-contract priority selection, then so be it.

Finally, Fitzroy relented. They could see me leaving the club for nothing, so they negotiated a deal in which Brisbane gave them David Bain, Nigel Palfreyman and their original first-round selection in the draft, pick No. 7. Ironically, this pick would turn out to be Jacana teenager Chris Johnson, who three years later would join me in Brisbane via the Brisbane–Fitzroy merger. But that was a long way down the track.

Not so far off was Nathan Buckley's switch from Brisbane to Collingwood. It was all over the media. The first thing I'd wanted to do when I'd committed to the Bears was call 'Bucks', just on the off chance that I might be able to convince him to stay. I knew the club had a fantastic young brigade, but the then 21-year-old midfielder, who had won the AFL's Rising Star Award in his first season and finished runner-up to Michael McLean in the Bears' best and fairest, would really have topped us off.

Who knows what might have happened if Buckley had stayed in Brisbane? But I was told by the club not to bother. The deal was done. Apparently it had been done long before the future Collingwood captain and Brownlow medallist even moved north.

We finished our Noosa holiday and then Peta and I, and the Blakeys, had a week at Palm Beach on the Gold Coast in an apartment owned by John Richmond, a Hobart football legend and owner of a pub where I'd put in a few hours behind the bar. It was there that I finally signed the paperwork for the trade from Fitzroy to Brisbane. Shane Johnson, Bears football manager and another proud Tasmanian, drove down from Brisbane with pen in hand. At last it was all official.

But it wasn't over. Not quite. There had been a lot of comment among Fitzroy supporters, and my old favourites, the Lynch Mob, had called a meeting at the Fitzroy Club Hotel in Northcote. I'm not quite sure what they were hoping to achieve, but I knew one thing — I had to go.

The Lynch Mob were my most passionate supporters. They were footy fanatics who struggled to find the money each year to buy their Fitzroy membership. Often, they went without things that should have been more important just so they could sit out in the wind and rain with their giant 'Lynch Mob' banner whenever Fitzroy played. They just loved their footy. Occasionally they'd even end up in a fight while defending the honour of their club, but they'd be back the next week regardless. They'd been fantastic to me since 1989 and I felt the least I could do was go and see them.

So, about 6pm, I walked unannounced into the hotel. Expecting a handful of people, I was astounded to find more like 400. And as fate would have it, the first people I saw were two young boys, Shane and Warwick, and their mother Rhonda, whom I'd been very close to throughout my time at the club. I'd given Warwick a tracksuit top as I walked off the ground after a game a few years earlier and they were incredibly loyal thereafter. They were in tears, saying, 'You can't go.' I knew it was going to be a tough night.

I got up on stage with the intention of explaining the reasons for my decision. I knew I wasn't going to appease them, such was their passion for Fitzroy, but I wanted to try to make them understand. Well, I couldn't speak. 'Give me a minute,' I said.

Having done my best to compose myself, I tried to explain my feelings for Fitzroy. How privileged I felt to have had six years at the club and what a tremendous bond I felt with all the people associated with the club. It was just something I had to do. And while I probably didn't ease the angst or disappointment much, a good number of them understood my situation.

I never went back to the club again. I was never with the Fitzroy players as an entire group again, although I spoke individually to most of them and caught up with many. That was what Fitzroy was about to me, the mateship. Long after we went our separate football ways we remained the closest of friends, often catching up for coffee, lunch, a game of golf or, out of season, a beer. Paul Roos, John Blakey, Paul Broderick, Matty Armstrong, Ross Lyon, Scott Clayton, Michael Gale, Darren Kappler and Duane Rowe. And others. It was a tragedy that one of Fitzroy's great strengths, the unique bond between the players, would survive longer than the club itself in its own right.

5

TROUBLE IN PARADISE

I awoke on Wednesday, 14 September 1994 lying flat on my back and feeling like I had a 100kg weight on my chest. I had shocking pains in my lower stomach, a throbbing headache and no energy. It was like the worst hangover I'd ever had, but worse. Getting out of bed was a monumental effort. And when I finally got to the bathroom my urine was pure black. Like ink. I knew something was wrong.

Two days earlier, on the Monday, I'd returned from the Brisbane Bears' end-of-season trip to Cairns. I was feeling pretty dusty, but that was to be expected. It had been a big weekend. Two pretty solid days and nights on the grog, including a day at the Cairns Amateurs races and a torturous day on the Great Barrier Reef. Tuesday, I was starting to feel better. But on the Wednesday it hit me. I was worse again. Much worse.

This was the beginning of the illness I later learned was chronic fatigue syndrome. An illness that would change my life forever. And the single reason I have written this book.

Season 1994 was my first with the Bears. After my much-publicised transfer from Fitzroy, it was to have been the start of an exciting new phase of my career. The best time of my life. However, it had turned into an unmitigated disaster. On and off the field.

Even my first training session with the club out at Queensland University was filled with drama. My back was really tight, and after a gentle warm-up we went into a 20m end-to-end handball drill. I'd deliberately done a couple of extra minutes of stretching and had the physiotherapist crack my back, but it was still pretty stiff. A 17-year-old Nigel Lappin, who hadn't been at the club much longer than I had, speared a firm handball above my head, and as I reached to grab it my back locked up and went into spasm. I hit the deck, and there I stayed for two or three minutes. I was staying with Peter Blucher, the club's communications manager, at the time, and as he drove me around for the next couple of days to inspect units Peta and I might move into I could do no more than lie across the back seat of the car.

I had also broken my collarbone twice. First in an intra-club practice match at Broadbeach which delayed my premiership debut for the club until Round 4. And then again in Round 17, which ended my season. And while I was recovering from that I also had to undergo surgery for a knee problem. It wasn't a good start. I'd played only 13 games, mainly at centre half forward, and we'd won only nine games and finished 12th out of 15 teams. Not the result we were looking for after a recruiting campaign which had also lured Craig Lambert, Andrew Bews, Gilbert McAdam, Craig Starcevich, Troy Lehmann and first-round draftees Nigel Lappin and Chris Scott to the club.

In something that's a bit strange, I didn't play in either of the two games against Fitzroy that year. My first Bears game, against St Kilda — I kicked a soft eight goals without leaving the goal square too often — was the week after the Bears played Fitzroy. And the game against Richmond in which I broke my collarbone the second time was the week before we played Fitzroy again. The only time I'd ever play against my old club was in a practice match at Queen Elizabeth Oval, Bendigo, in 1995; I didn't do too much damage because I was still asleep, but a young fella called Chris Johnson kicked four goals for Fitzroy, who won by 12 points.

But the 1994 disappointment wasn't only about football. We'd also had a burglary at home, a car accident and a death in the family.

Peta and I were living in a second-floor apartment at Auchenflower, overlooking Coronation Drive and the Brisbane River. We were robbed on the Thursday night before my second game with the club, which was a Friday night match against Melbourne at the MCG. It was a wet night and the road below could be a bit noisy in the rain, so we slept in a back room. We'd left the dryer on and so, to ensure some air circulation, we'd also left a kitchen window open. While we slept, someone climbed up the outside of the building and broke in. We never caught him, but we knew he was a smoker because he left cigarette ash in the unit. He took only small things — watches, jewellery, CDs and loose change — but it was terribly disconcerting to think that someone had been in our unit while we were asleep. Just as disconcerting for me was the fact that I had to fly to Melbourne first thing the next morning. Peta, still pretty much a stranger in town, would be left on her own. Happily, Terry and Shirl Hehir, friends we'd known from Melbourne who had been living in Brisbane for a couple of years, invited Pete to spend the night with them.

Not long afterwards, although very much a minor thing in comparison with what was to come, I was involved in a car accident. I'd left my car with Toowong Mitsubishi to get serviced. Terry Hehir, the manager, was good enough to lend me a car for the day: a brand new Prado. I drove to training at the Gabba and was heading back to Toowong along Coronation Drive when the two cars in front of me were involved in a nose-to-tail. I stopped short of them, but two cars behind me didn't. They ploughed into the back of the Prado. I'd had it five hours and managed to inflict $3000 worth of damage! Not my fault, and fortunately Terry was very good about it, but it was definitely something I could have done without.

Later, in July, Pete, who was working for a travel agency, had taken a tour group to the World Cup soccer tournament in the United States. Two days before she was due home, her stepfather Barry Joel had called me with the shattering news that Pete's mother Karen had cancer.

We felt there wasn't anything to be gained by telling Pete while she was away, so we waited until she got home on the Wednesday. Her mother, already suffering badly with arthritis, was very weak, so Pete booked a trip to Melbourne for the following weekend. Her mother was to have her first round of chemotherapy on the Friday but she died that day. It was 22 July, a sad, sad day for us all.

I was working with Coca-Cola at the time and was scheduled to play golf that day but I decided to cancel and go home to spend time with Peta. Not long afterwards Peta's stepfather called to say Karen had gone. I can still hear Pete's words: 'Where's she gone? What do you mean she's gone?'

Karen hadn't got through the chemotherapy. I couldn't help but think how fortunate it was that I wasn't off playing golf, uncontactable for several hours, having left Pete to not only take the phone call but deal with the devastating news by herself. Still settling into Brisbane, without any really close friends nearby, it would have been even worse than the heartbreak it was.

The news was shattering. Pete was so close to her mum. Leaving Melbourne had been really hard for her because they were such a close family, especially mother and daughter. Karen would often invite me round for a mid-morning cup of tea and cake when we lived close by in Melbourne. She was so easy to talk to and very proud of her kids.

What hurts terribly is that Karen didn't live to share the most important moments in her daughter's life. She missed our wedding, and all the fuss and preparation needed to make sure her daughter's special day was perfect. Just seeing her walk down the aisle would have been such a thrill. And she missed the birth of our children. Madison would have been her first grandchild. We had often told Karen that we liked that name, after meeting ex-Fitzroy teammate Gavin Exell's daughter Madison. So that was it. We couldn't change it.

All in all, it had been a miserable year. So, having undergone my knee surgery, I headed to Cairns looking to wipe the slate clean; to officially close season 1994 and begin afresh for 1995. It was a terrific weekend. I was still getting to know my new teammates and wanted to make the most of it. We had a great holiday although I could have done without the day when 20-odd blokes, feeling less than well, had the time from hell on the reef. The seas were rough and the boat kept rocking and rocking and rocking. Not good for a hangover. People were sick everywhere, and not just because of the night before. It was a shocking day. Damian Bourke, ex-Geelong captain turned Brisbane ruckman, and Wayne Brittain, Bears assistant coach and later coach of Carlton, were prepared to pay virtually anything for a helicopter to airlift them to dry land. I would happily have gone too.

All of these things meant I wasn't totally surprised that I was unwell when we flew home to Brisbane on the Monday. Even that I was still a bit off on the Tuesday. But Wednesday was the killer. Aches and pains like I'd never felt before. Peta took me to a doctor, and a few days later, after a range of blood tests, he told me I'd had some form of viral infection and would come good in a few days.

I didn't. I got worse, much worse. I saw a specialist at the Wesley Hospital. More blood tests. Same diagnosis. Same prognosis. Give it time, they said. Nothing else we can do.

Time! I had plenty of that. I was sleeping 18 hours a day. I'd struggle to get up with Peta in the morning, and occasionally I'd have some breakfast. When she went to work, I went back to bed. The next thing I knew was when she got home, around six o'clock. Maybe a little dinner and television, and then I was off to bed again. This was how I spent much of October 1994. My energy levels fluctuated. Sometimes it wasn't that bad. On the good days I felt as if I had a hangover or flu. A headache and a mind which was permanently cloudy. Summer training had begun in late October, and on the good days I'd try to train. After all, I was the so-called boom recruit. I couldn't be sitting around idle. The medical fraternity had told me that although they couldn't do anything for me, there was nothing seriously wrong and I'd get better in time. But the pressure, more from within than from anywhere else, was mounting. I'd had an injury-disrupted first season with the Bears. I had to get myself fit and ready for the start of 1995.

It was the worst thing I could have done. Every time I'd push myself, it would set me back even further. I got into the vicious circle of spending long days in bed, then when I felt better I'd train. Then I'd have a relapse. The frustration was incredible. There I was, an athlete in the prime of my career, barely able to get out of bed. And nobody could tell me why. Worse still, they couldn't give me any indication of when I would feel better. I was doing what they told me to do. I was taking a whole range of supplements that were meant to help make my body healthy enough to fix itself. But it wasn't working.

The illness had become a hot topic in the media. It wasn't glandular fever or Ross River fever, as was suggested, so they called it a mystery virus. A good media term. Whatever it was, it not only took me out of football, it took away my social life. Virtually every hour was spent within the four walls of our two-bedroom apartment. We were unable to socialise, or to consolidate friendships in a still unfamiliar city.

I tried everything. More doctors and specialists than you can imagine. A daily one-hour stint in a hyperbaric chamber. A two-hour intravenous drip twice a week. More supplements. And when traditional medicine failed me I looked elsewhere. I tried naturopaths, chiropractors, holistic medicine and a few people on the Gold Coast I can't begin to describe. One group had me sitting down holding a steel rod that was connected to a computer watching colourful patterns on the screen while listening to music. It was supposed to help my body rhythms, but I'd categorise it under the 'load of rubbish' banner. But I was so desperate for answers that I was willing to try it.

In Brisbane I'd even been sent by the Bears club doctor Alan Mackenzie for a psychiatric assessment at the Princess Alexandra Hospital on Ipswich Road, not far from the Gabba. There, a specialist asked questions about my relationship with my father. I was open to anything if they could prove it, but I knew this was another load of rubbish. I was depressed, certainly. Very much so. Because

I didn't know what was wrong or when I'd get better. But I knew that the depression wasn't the underlying cause.

It was a horrendous period, and, as I've said over and over again, I wouldn't have got through it without Peta. At the time it was all about me, yet 10 years on I still marvel at how she coped. So, to complete the picture and provide her perspective on this living nightmare, we sat down in a formal interview situation and she recounted her memories. I'll let her tell her story.

'My recollections and emotions were the same as Alastair's because we were in it together. We weren't close to many people in Brisbane, certainly not in the way we were close to our friends in Melbourne, and all of a sudden, because of his illness, we were even more isolated. We pretty much had each other.

'We'd both led a pretty charmed life up until this point — he'd only ever missed two games of football in the time I'd known him before we left Fitzroy. I didn't want to move to Brisbane — I was happy to go because it was what he had to do and it was a fantastic opportunity — but if it was just my decision we would have stayed in Melbourne with family and friends.

'First things started to go wrong with his football and then my mum died in July 1994. And then in September

1994 he went to Cairns and came back sick. All of a sudden we were in a different world — our own little insular world.

'How did I feel? Confused, frustrated — I felt everything he felt. What is it? Why is he sick? When would he get better? Would he get better? The fact that it came out of nowhere without warning and turned our entire life upside down made me feel so helpless, yet I knew I had to be positive. I couldn't afford to let it get on top of me because that wasn't going to help him get better.

'It was a bizarre existence — watching him drink olive oil and throw up because somebody said it might be good for him, and growing this mushroom-type fungus in the fridge because it may have some healing qualities. I felt like his doctor some days, even though I had no idea what I was doing. We just had to do what we had to do. I would have done anything to make him better, yet one of the best things I could do for him was buy him a couple of bags of ice so he could jump in his iced bath.

'I never doubted for one second that he was sick — it was right there in front of me every day — but I guess there was probably a time when even I wondered if it was all in his head because so many people were saying that. They'd say, "Why can't he just go out and try to play?" and until we knew the cause of it all you couldn't blame them. The uncertainty of it all was the worst part.

'I was very worried about him for a while. I don't know that I ever thought he'd jump off the bridge or anything like that, but I guess the fact that I even mention that tells me that sort of thing must have crossed my mind. It was such a mental challenge to get on top of it all and I always felt we had to conquer that before we could tackle the physical challenge. He had to believe he was going to get better.

'I leaned very heavily on family and friends, especially my dad and Sharlene Broderick [wife of former Fitzroy and Richmond footballer Paul Broderick] — there were a lot of long phone calls to Melbourne from that poky little unit at Auchenflower. Without them I wouldn't have got through it. "Sharles" was an absolute rock — she rode it with me, she never doubted us for one second and was never anything but 100 per cent supportive, which was exactly what I needed.

'I was also lucky to have my job at Travelworld at South Brisbane because that gave me another outlet and something to do rather than just worrying about him.

'It was the weirdest, most distressing time of my life and I couldn't have done it forever. If it had continued I would have had to go home to Melbourne. We were only in Brisbane for Al to play football and I couldn't have coped indefinitely, but thankfully it never got to the stage where going home was at the forefront of my mind.

'What did the whole experience do for us? It made us a better couple because we only had each other. It was something we had to battle through together, and it made us appreciate something simple like your health which for so long we took for granted.

'I don't think I'll ever be totally convinced that he's over it because there are still times when he gets run down. I'll always have that fear in the back of my mind.

'I'd never want him to be sick but it's given us a different perspective on things and to come back and do the whole football thing after what he went through is terribly satisfying. The first grand final when the siren went and he had the ball in his hands — that was the moment for me. It made everything all worthwhile.'

But the 2001 grand final was still an eternity away. Nothing much changed through November and December 1994. Christmas in Melbourne with Peta's family was a write-off. More of the same in January. But what could I do? There was supposedly nothing wrong with me. When I was able to I kept training. Especially after a specialist diagnosed chronic sinusitis. Perhaps this was the answer.

In the meantime I saw other specialists who suggested CMV: cytomegolovirus infection. My research told me that this was a virus most frequently transmitted to a developing child before birth, and that it was known to infect upwards of half the population by the age of 40. For most healthy people who acquire CMV after birth there are few symptoms and no long-term consequences. A small minority experience a mononucleosis-like syndrome with prolonged fever, and a mild hepatitis. Usually, though, the virus, while still alive, remains dormant within that person's body for life. So for the vast majority, CMV infection is not a serious problem. Maybe I was the exception. Part of me hoped I was. At least then I'd have an answer. But there was no medical evidence to support this. We still didn't know what was wrong.

In February 1995 I played a couple of practice matches, and in Round 1 of the premiership I kicked two goals against Hawthorn at Waverley, but I was still feeling dreadful. It was just so frustrating, for me and for the club. I could understand that. They had a vice-captain who was supposed to help turn the club around, and he was currently almost completely unproductive.

I guess it could have been worse: I could have been captain. And in fact I could have been — the club had offered me the captaincy when they were attempting to lure me to Brisbane, but I had declined. Roger Merrett had been Bears captain since 1990, and the last thing I wanted to do was upset the status quo. My time would come if it was meant to be, and if not it didn't matter. There was never anything in writing, despite what I read many times over the years, and I was happy always to be judged on merit.

I couldn't help feeling that there was nevertheless a little uncertainty towards me from Roger from the start. The club had made a huge fuss about signing me and had immediately made me the face of their marketing. I suspected that the captain might feel I hadn't earned my stripes, and that it had all come too easily. I could sympathise with them, but realistically what could I do? The club wanted to capitalise on its 10-year investment and I could hardly say no. No doubt when I got sick, the uncertainty grew. And fair enough. I didn't understand what was going on so I could hardly expect others to do so. The players were very good to my face, but sometimes I wondered what might have been said behind my back. I couldn't blame them if they found it all a bit too much. It was a difficult time for us all.

In the end, we lost to Hawthorn by 57 points in Round 1 on 1 April. On the following Monday we had a big running session at the Gabba. Mainly 200m and 400m runs. I couldn't complete the session. I was feeling dizzy and lethargic. As if I was going to fall over all the time. This wasn't just me unfit and fatigued. It was more than that. I could see myself crashing back to the worst days of a few months earlier.

Via my manager, Damien Smith, I got an appointment to see Melbourne ear, nose and throat specialist Dr Jack Kennedy. He was a Collingwood man and was renowned in AFL circles. He was to address my recently diagnosed sinus problems and, through his extensive network of colleagues, to eliminate as many conditions as possible in order to find out what was wrong. I spent three days in Melbourne, staying with my ex-Fitzroy teammate John Blakey, while seeing a range of people. I had yet more blood tests, scans for brain tumours and an AIDS test. A second one. Not even when I told them I'd already had this done in Brisbane would they desist. So I did it all. My lymph glands were swollen, so I went to see an oncologist. Word spread quickly. A League footballer visiting a cancer specialist doesn't stay secret for long in Melbourne, and while I was on a plane flying back to Brisbane, Peta's father, Neil, rang her to say the media was carrying a story that I had cancer. You can imagine how well that went down. Peta couldn't even contact me so that I could put her mind at ease.

Jack Kennedy determined, through this process of elimination, that I had post-viral syndrome. Or chronic fatigue syndrome (CFS), as it had occasionally been called and which would become the popular name. He ordered me to rest and stressed the importance of doing as he instructed. Failure to rest adequately, he said, could have dire consequences. It could mean that I'd be plagued by this condition for the rest of my life. It could cost me my career, he warned. He wrote to the club explaining the seriousness of the situation, but at this stage I wasn't worrying about my career. I just wanted to get healthy.

Dr Kennedy, a wonderful support at a crucial time, in fact wrote three letters of significance. On 18 April 1995 he wrote to Dr Alan Mackenzie of the Bears advising that I'd seen Dr Newton Lee, haematologist and oncologist, and Dr John Niall, renal physician. He advised against the sinus surgery that was being considered at the time, and recommended to the club that I not engage in any form of training for at least a month. He encouraged me to undertake some casual activity like golf and limited exercise like tennis, and indicated he would see me again in a month.

On 9 May 1995, after a follow-up visit, he wrote to Scott Clayton at the Bears and told Scott how, even after having a kick of the football a week earlier, I'd become quite fatigued. He wrote: 'He still needs one more month off full training and . . . I have told him that he is not to be playing any football or taking part in any rigorous training programs in this time.'

And, on 17 July 1995, Dr Kennedy wrote to Dr Peter Harcourt, then at the Victorian Institute of Sport, after I'd been sent there as part of the rehabilitation process. He explained to Dr Harcourt, later to play a more pivotal role in a much bigger matter, the background to my illness and wrote: 'I have seen him on three occasions and have recommended that he should not be going back to training and football at all this year because when he did attempt to do this, against advice, he became fatigued again.'

So rest I did, and slowly I improved. But I made a mistake. Feeling indebted to the club, I made sure I was around the place as much as possible. I was forever being asked questions I couldn't answer. And by visiting the club regularly I created the myth that there was nothing seriously wrong. To those who didn't know, I looked fine.

Still, feeling a little better I began walking a couple of laps, just to get the body going a little, and it created an expectation that I was on the mend. I should have stayed away.

By mid-1995, although I'd ruled out the possibility of playing football again that season, I was at least heading in the right direction. It was two steps forward, one step back, though. Sometimes three steps back. I was frustrated by the rate of improvement. It was all happening too slowly. So I continued looking for answers.

I rang Barry Sheene, the 1976–77 500cc world motorcycle champion who lived on the Gold Coast. He was one of the few CFS patients who had publicly discussed his condition. I had a long phone conversation with him and he was magnificent. He understood exactly the frustration I was feeling, and among other things, he recommended ice baths. They had worked so successfully for him that he'd installed a spa at his home with a connection to an air-conditioner to regulate the temperature. By now it was midwinter, and the pool at our apartment building was perfect. In the early morning it was 11°C. So each day I'd get up at 8am and sit in the cold pool for 20 minutes, sometimes longer. Bears fitness coach Craig Maskiell, a top triathlete who was studying medicine at the time and is now a doctor at Nambour Hospital, came and sat with me a couple of times. All because he wanted to offer support and better understand what I was going through. But he was so lean that he couldn't stand the cold.

I loved the cold baths. Essentially, it was one big adrenaline rush — no different from what anyone gets when they jump into icy cold water. The difference was that for the next two or three hours I felt some relief. So I did it every day, sometimes twice a day, for eight months. When summer came and the pool wasn't cold enough, I'd simulate the same thing in the bath. In the spare fridge we'd keep a few big blocks of ice, or Peta would pick up some from the local service station or the bottle shop. I felt stupid, but I used to really look forward to it because it made me feel better for a while. And I hadn't felt good for a long time.

I developed an enormous regard for Barry Sheene. He'd found a way to get on top of his CFS and he was only too happy to share his experience. I talked to him often when he wasn't jet-setting around the world, and after a while not always about CFS, because we shared a love of sport. A couple of years later, when I was in the studios of Brisbane radio station B105FM doing a breakfast interview, he called the station. 'Ali,' he said, as he used to call me. 'I'm really, really stuffed. Have you found anything new that you can help me with?' He'd suffered a relapse and was now seeking the same sort of assistance he'd offered me. Sadly, there wasn't a lot I could do. Especially when he was diagnosed with cancer in July 2002. It was one of my enormous regrets that when he died in March 2003, aged 52, I'd never met him face to face.

Around the time I started with the ice baths, Robert Walls, probably almost as frustrated as I was, arranged for me to see a friend of his at Pottsville, on the northern NSW coast. Maurie Rayner, who later died of cancer, was originally from the Bells Beach–Torquay area of Victoria. He was well known as a surf lifesaver/ironman, and had a health resort at Bellbrae, down on the Great Ocean Road. He had been fitness coach under Wallsy at Fitzroy in 1981–82, and Wallsy thought he might be able to help me, so Peta and I headed south to Pottsville one Friday afternoon mid-year. Pete was only going to stay for a day, but I was booked in for the weekend at a private home with a magnificent outlook, right on the Pacific Ocean.

We had a lovely dinner on the Friday night with Maurie and his wife. We spoke a little about my problem and about goal-setting. He had us cut out some pictures from newspapers and magazines which were supposed to represent where we wanted to be in life. We went to bed more than a little puzzled. Next thing I knew it was about 5.30am and I heard a voice outside my window saying — twice — 'Alastair, it's time to get up.' I had no idea what was going on, but as instructed, I dragged on some shorts and a T-shirt. I was off for a run and a paddle.

Maurie had two big Malibu boards. That was one each. The surf was really gentle, but I struggled to paddle through it. Every time I'd take a stroke forward, my other arm struggled to raise out of the water. Finally, we were beyond the beach break and headed north. We didn't get far when finally he got the message. I was spent. We went back in and took the boards home. A rest, I thought. Not at all. He'd set up a mini weights circuit with small dumbbells. Again, I was struggling. He gave me an odd look and said, 'You're not as strong as you look.' I was staggered. 'Go on,' I said to him, before explaining once again my ongoing battle.

It was a bizarre experience. Pete had to get back to Brisbane; as I learned later, she cried almost the whole way home. She was worried I'd be pushed too hard, confused as to why the club had sent me down to do training sessions I couldn't get through. I stayed for the rest of the weekend, but there wasn't a lot of physical activity after Maurie realised I couldn't tolerate it. We talked a lot and he grilled me about my attitudes to life. He even had me doing some deep-breathing exercises. The more he went on, the more confused I became. A couple of weeks later he came to Brisbane for a further meeting with Robert Walls and me. It became evident that he thought our relationship was struggling, but that wasn't true. I had nothing but total respect for Wallsy. Sure, we'd had a difference of opinion in 1994 over my allegiance to some of my ex-Fitzroy teammates, but we'd agreed to disagree on that one and moved on. No doubt Wallsy was struggling with the fact that I wasn't able to play football, but that was a result of my illness, not a cause.

When I was putting this book together, I thought it would be interesting to ask Robert Walls to reflect on his two years as my coach in Brisbane, and it was. As always, Wallsy didn't pull any punches.

'I was just so very, very frustrated and disappointed for the player and the club. He'd come up on a big long-term deal worth lots of money and there were massive hopes. He was the club's biggest signing since Roger Merrett in 1988, and it had been a long time since we'd landed a really big fish. We'd tried a few like Jason Dunstall without any success and everyone was really excited that this guy was going to help turn things around. In my first two or three years (1991–92–93) we'd only ever been expected to win four games, but now we were setting the bar a lot higher — in 1994 we had to be looking for something like a break-even result,' he said.

'He broke his collarbone twice in his first year in Brisbane [1994] — that was disappointing but it happens. And then for him to get sick, well, it was just the double whammy. We couldn't take a trick.

'I shared the frustration that he felt because nobody could give us any answers. Sometimes he'd look OK and other times he was flat as a tack. One minute I was optimistic and the next minute I was pessimistic. Even if somebody could have said he'd be right to go in 10 weeks I would have been happy. That's half a season and a long time in football, but we couldn't even get that out of anyone.'

Did he ever question my commitment to Brisbane? 'I never doubted his commitment to the club but I did get to the stage where I wondered if it was more mental than physical. I thought maybe it was all playing on his mind. He'd left a club where he was very popular and things were going well. He was cruising. Then, to come to

Brisbane, he was the focus of all the attention. He was the great white hope and expectations were huge. He'd never experienced anything like that before so it was new territory,' said Wallsy.

'I'd really admired the way he'd come back from his broken collarbone. When it happened the medical staff told me what a dreadful injury it is because it really knocks a player's confidence around, but he got through that pretty well and played some really good football in '94. And then '95 he couldn't play.

'When I left Brisbane I thought the club had done its dough. I just couldn't see it working. I watched his progress very closely and to be honest he had to play three years of really good football for me to say maybe it will work after all.

'Well, he did much more than that. He played 11 years and was just a wonderful player, and not only did he do it on the field but was really good for the club off the field, too. I salute him and I take my hat off to him. I respect greatly what he's done. He had to earn my respect the hard way and he did that.

'It's fair to say our relationship by the end of the two years wasn't strong because it wasn't built on anything. But now it's very good and I'm very happy about that.'

Scott Clayton, a former Fitzroy teammate and good friend turned Brisbane Bears director of football, had played a huge role in getting me to Brisbane and was one of my closest confidants during this horrendous time.

He's now recruiting manager at the Western Bulldogs, building an exciting young team just as he did in Brisbane. I asked him, too, to revisit my first couple of years with the Bears through his eyes. He was predictably loyal, as he'd always been.

He said: 'Looking back on it I wonder what else we could have done to help ... I feel we as a club let him down a little bit because we couldn't offer anything more than moral support. But it was such a difficult thing because we didn't have any answers. In the early stages maybe we erred by saying to the media, "We think he'll be right in a couple of weeks", and then "He should be back in three weeks", when really all we were doing was hoping. We didn't know. Maybe this created an unreal expectation and put more pressure on him. I know one thing for certain — if the same thing happened today at an AFL club they'd do it better because the system is more conscious of these sorts of issues and much better-equipped to handle them.

'I got disappointed when I heard people question Lynchy's commitment to the club because those who really knew him knew this was never, ever an issue — not at all. I can understand because the frustration got to everyone, but he couldn't have been more committed to the Brisbane Football Club. It was as if he was trying to pull himself over the top of a hedge — he'd take one small step at a time and just when he was starting to make some headway a limb would keep breaking. He was trying so hard. In fact, maybe this was part of the problem — he tried too hard to get back too quickly when he should have taken a longer period of time just to make sure he was right.

'But it's all just speculation because the fact of the matter was nobody knew the best way to handle it. All I know is that he was one very sick man — gaunt, white, grey even. He just looked terribly ill. I remember walking a couple of laps of the Gabba with him a few times when he started to get a little better, bouncing the ball and talking as we went. We'd even had a few kicks but that was all he could manage. I felt helpless because I felt I should have been able to do more for him. At that stage football wasn't even a consideration. We just wanted him to get back some sort of normal health.'

In fact, it was people like Scott who really helped me through the tough times because I knew his support was unconditional. I knew that he would back me to the hilt, and that was terribly important.

Exactly what the other players were saying was more difficult for me to know. As I said, nobody was ever anything but totally supportive to my face, but I had to wonder if privately some players weren't questioning what was going on. And who could blame them? Not me. Not when I was going through the same frustration and uncertainty.

In the interests of providing a more comprehensive feel for the mood of the team during my illness, and at the risk of being embarrassed, I've given a couple of former teammates a chance to have their say.

Trent Bartlett was a big, raw-boned teenager from Deloraine in northern Tasmania who had joined the Bears at the same time as me in 1994. He made his AFL debut in the year I missed through illness and played a total of 39 games for the Bears from 1995 to 1999, including the club's first final in September '95, before playing 36 games with the Western Bulldogs in 2000–01. He lived on my side of town and, being a fellow Tasmanian, I felt a certain connection and even a responsibility to help him. We were always good mates.

He said: 'I'm embarrassed even to be asked about Lynchy because as a kid I had a poster of him on my bedroom wall. He was the Tasmanian idol at Fitzroy when I was growing up and next thing I know I'm drafted by the Bears and he's recruited as the gun. It was a weird feeling. But he and Peta looked after me incredibly well — I reckon I had dinner at their home just about every Wednesday night for two years.

'It was a standing invitation but I didn't feel comfortable going when I knew he was crook. Sometimes I'd get there after training about seven o'clock and he'd still be in bed. Other times he'd try to pretend he'd cooked dinner but I always knew it was Peta. And then after dinner I'd be talking to Peta, and Lynchy would quietly take himself back to bed because he couldn't stay awake any longer. I didn't quite know how to handle it because I was just a kid living my football dream, and to see one of the all-time greats struggling so badly was terrible. It didn't seem fair. We had a lot of young players and I reckon they felt the same way. I can't speak for the entire group but I think most guys just felt a mixture of sympathy and frustration for him,' said 'Bart', now filling a key football administration role with AFL Tasmania, looking after the representative teams.

Nigel Lappin was another player who had been drafted to the Bears in 1994. Unlike Bart, who had to earn his stripes, Nige pretty much went straight into the senior side in his first season. It was the beginning of a career that would top 250-plus games in Brisbane and include three premierships and untold individual awards. Yet he never changed from the quiet, shy boy from Chiltern in north-eastern Victoria.

In late 1994 and early 1995, when I was working at the club in a marketing role, Nige was doing a hospitality traineeship at the Bears Social Club. So we'd often have lunch together.

He said: 'I've got a vivid recollection of a day in my first year when Wallsy asked me to play golf with Lynchy and 'Choppers' [Marcus Ashcroft] at Surfers Paradise. For a kid like me who was in awe of the coach and the senior players it was incredible. Afterwards Lynchy invited me back to his place. We had a hit of tennis on the court at the apartment block where he was living and then I stayed for dinner with him and Peta. It was like I'd known them for 20 years and I felt bad when I had to leave. That sort of thing was such a thrill for a young kid back then and it doesn't seem to happen as much these days.

'Lynchy had played some great games for the club in 1994 in between his two broken collarbones and when he got sick I couldn't believe it. It was just such a tragedy because he was in the prime of his career and we could have become a successful side much earlier than we eventually were if he'd stayed on the field.

'I'd see him around the club during the day and he'd look terrible. I'd go downstairs and he'd be half asleep at his desk, and other times you'd find him having a cold bath down in the footy rooms.

'I never really understood what he was going through even though I felt so sorry for him. I remember one day at training at the University of Queensland, so it must have been early '95, and he and Doc Mackenzie [club doctor Alan Mackenzie] were giving the players an update. He told us it was a sinus problem and I just thought great — he'll get it fixed and be back in a few weeks. That's the sort of mentality you had at that age. You were just caught up in your own little world having fun playing footy and trying to make a decent job of it.

'A bit later on, Doc and Lynchy gave us another update. They were standing out in front of the group and even though Lynchy was a very strong person you could see it was taking its toll on him. It was starting to get him down. I don't think too many of the younger guys understood it. You just expect him to have that invincibility about him and it was only as time went on and they were able to give us some concrete answers that we realised it was much more serious than that,' said Nigel.

I was pleased to learn from Michael Voss that he didn't think there was a lot of ill feeling among the playing group over my illness.

'There was certainly a lot of frustration and uncertainty about the whole thing, but there was no way I ever doubted him. The players as a group were just desperate to get him back because we knew he was among the best players in the competition and that at his best he'd make us better,' said Vossy.

'Looking back on it now, you realise just what he went through as a virtual pioneer for CFS in Australia. He had issues — no doubt about that. He'd turn up to a weights session with his eyeballs hanging out or embedded in the back of his head but the thing I admire most about Lynchy, over and above everything he achieved, was the fact that not once did he complain about it.'

In mid-July 1995, Bears director of football Scott Clayton received a phone call from Dr John Whiting. He was doing an extensive study of CFS patients throughout Australia and offered to help. It was good of him, because his books were closed. He was seeing so many CFS patients, and having some real success with them, that ordinarily new patients just couldn't get in. He made an exception for me.

Dr Whiting was born in Canada, raised in Ireland and moved to Australia in 1980. He had suffered from CFS himself, or at least a condition he later knew to be CFS, from the age of 12. He had a background in infectious diseases and microbiology. My first appointment with him was on 18 July. It was the first of 24 one-hour sessions over the next 12 months. And I would consult with him over the phone until March 1999.

Dr Whiting was the first doctor who could show me actual tests that proved my deficiencies. I didn't need to be convinced, but it was good to be able to show some sort of tangible proof to people at the club. That's why I'm tired and dizzy, I could say to them. That's why my energy levels and blood pressure are so low. For months I had weekly and sometimes bi-weekly blood tests, as Dr Whiting searched for trends and patterns in the irregularities in my immune system.

Scotty and Craig Maskiell came with me to some of my early appointments with Dr Whiting in his Wickham Terrace clinic. I'll never forget one session during which I just had to stand still while he measured various things. I lasted about 90 seconds before I blacked out. Just standing still I would quickly get dizzy and had to sit down. At least then I knew I wasn't the only person at the club who thought I was sick.

6

CFS: LIVING WITH IT

It was one thing for me to have CFS and to live with it and its complications and frustrations. But it was another thing for one of my best mates to see first-hand what it was all about, and just how debilitating it was. Public understanding and perception of CFS was always an issue. In the early days nobody really understood what it was, and many people doubted the illness really even existed. That was terribly frustrating, and certainly didn't help my situation.

There I was, a professional footballer of 26, in the prime of my career, with a team and a club that was on the climb, struggling to get out of bed. And people said there was nothing wrong with me. It just didn't add up. I'd made a difficult decision to move from Melbourne to Brisbane and it was potentially an exciting time. The prospect of playing a key role in a successful club was what my career was all about, but because of my illness I wasn't able to capitalise on any of it. So I'll never forget the look on Paul Roos' face when we walked into a chronic fatigue syndrome clinic in Los Angeles.

It was an early morning in October 1996. Peta and I had gone to visit Roosy and his wife Tami at Tami's family home in Saratoga, about 80km south of San Francisco. It was a dual-purpose holiday: to see our close friends and to visit world-acclaimed CFS specialist Dr Jay Goldstein, a director at the Chronic Fatigue Institute of Orange, California, and a professor at UCLA. Roosy, an inspiration and teammate in my early football career, then an opposition player and now senior coach of the Sydney Swans, generously offered to make the trip with me to Los Angeles. We caught a plane from Saratoga to John Wayne Airport in LA and stayed overnight outside Anaheim before my appointment the next day. As we entered the clinic his jaw hit the floor.

There were about half a dozen people of varying ages in the waiting room and every one of them was asleep. They were much worse affected than I had ever been. We sat and waited for a while and I could tell it had blown him away. There was a beautiful young girl in her early 20s. She had the head bobs going. She'd wake up and try to stay awake, but she just couldn't. Her head was bobbing up and down uncontrollably. The nurse had asked her to complete some registration forms but she wasn't even able to get up and walk across the room to the counter. Even when the nurse gave her the forms she struggled to fill them in, falling asleep between words.

The visit to Dr Goldstein was mainly to see if my treatment matched what he was prescribing — with excellent results — in the US. I wanted an expert second opinion. We'd sent him a copy of my files and he'd spoken at length with Dr John Whiting, my Brisbane specialist. He did some further blood tests, and everything stacked up, which was reassuring. But what was more important for me was just having a good friend see it all. It meant that I had someone more than my earbashed wife to discuss it with. Someone who actually knew what I was on about. Who wasn't just trying to be interested and understanding but really had a full appreciation of what an impact CFS could have. As Roosy said, it's like getting a hole in one playing golf by yourself — it's no good because you've got nobody to talk to about it.

If there's one word to describe the mixture of feelings that goes with CFS, or myalgic encephalomyelitis (ME), as it is known in many parts of the world, it is frustration. The uncertainty of it all is the killer. What causes it? How to treat it? And how long will it last? Give me a knee reconstruction over CFS any day. Because, as serious as a knee reconstruction is for a sportsman, at least it is a familiar and finite condition. Everyone knows what it is and how to remedy it. And you have a reasonable expectation that within 12 months, sometimes less, you will be fully fit and ready to resume competition. A knee injury only upsets your football — it doesn't turn your entire life upside down.

I don't know for sure what caused my CFS. All I have is a theory. I believe it may have been cumulative, where lots of things happened, one after the other, to wear my system down enough for it to be susceptible to infection. Certainly, 1994 had been a very stressful time. There was the decision to leave Fitzroy and move to Brisbane, the pre-season collarbone injury, the robbery, the death of Peta's mother, the car accident, the second collarbone injury and finally the knee operation. So when I went to Cairns for the end-of-season trip, which I'd specifically marked as a whole new beginning, perhaps I was vulnerable. I was worn out, and picked up a virus which my system didn't have the resources to fight off. It makes sense to me, and in the absence of any more definite medical theory, that's the one I go with.

The failure of some doctors to recognise CFS is also hugely frustrating. One doctor I saw several times began our first consultation with, 'I don't believe in CFS but I'm going to find out what's causing your problems!' He conceded, at least, that there was something wrong with me, which was more than some had done. It was too easy to say 'It's a virus — you'll be right soon.'

The 'it's all in the head' theory was pretty common in the early days of my illness, and pretty disheartening. I would say to people, 'Why wouldn't I want to be healthy?' To me it was just inconceivable that I would choose to be ill. But as time wore on, and nobody could give me any concrete answers, I did start to wonder. In the end it didn't matter. If it is a psychological condition, give me something to rectify it, I'd say. If it's a physical problem, fix it. I didn't care. I just wanted some answers.

I saw somewhere between 30 and 40 medical practitioners, ranging from accredited specialists to what might commonly be called 'witch doctors'. As time went on and traditional medicine couldn't find a cure, I was prepared to try anything. Dr Jack Kennedy's diagnosis in April 1995 was a key time. So, too, was the beginning of my association with Dr Whiting. They gave me something to hang on to. A reason to believe that I could and would get better.

A University of Newcastle research program which I was introduced to through Dr Whiting was also a big positive for me. Their four-man team targeted not just CFS, but also other related conditions, such as fibromyalgia, rheumatoid arthritis, chronic pain and tempero mandibular joint dysfunction. The team was Associate Professors Dr Hugh Dunstan and Dr Tim Roberts, microbiologist Dr Henry Butt, and local dentist Dr Neil McGregor. I cannot say categorically that they are right — only history and an all-encompassing cure for CFS will be the final judge of that — but what they said at the time (and continue to say) made good sense to a layman, so I was happy to work with them.

It was through this study that I learned of Dr Cecile Jadin, who had studied in Belgium and worked extensively in South Africa. Her theory on managing CFS, which had been tried with some success in South Africa, was a 12-month program of antibiotics. So I flew to Newcastle to visit a doctor who, working on the same philosophy, prescribed a 12-month revolving cycle of antibiotics. Did it help? I cannot be sure. But it certainly didn't hurt and I was prepared to try anything that came well recommended.

The Newcastle team was broken up in 2001, and only Dr Roberts and Dr Dunstan continue their research there, but it was then and still is their belief that CFS is caused by an ongoing infection in which bacteria live in the cells of the body.

When you have an acute infection, which can be as simple as flu or a severe poisoning, your temperature goes up and your system wants to shut down. You go off your food, want to sit quietly, not talk to anyone and do nothing. Pretty much just sleep. That is your body marshalling its troops to begin the defence process. But if in this process you are breaking down your own protein supplies, then you are effectively losing muscle tone and body weight. If you can't clear the infection, eventually your entire system becomes dysfunctional. You become malnourished, are short on amino acids and essential fatty acids, and your adrenal glands stop doing their job properly, causing fatigue.

According to the Newcastle research crew, this also involves the biochemical pathway which converts cholesterol into progesterone. Progesterone is then converted into three things: glucocorticoid (which looks after the immune system), testosterone and DHEA (produced by the adrenal glands and which act to prevent fatigue), and mineralcorticoid (which impacts on blood pressure).

All three of these factors are directly related to CFS. The research team has found that the bulk of CFS sufferers have low blood pressure, low testosterone and DHEA, and have variable levels of glucocorticoid. Essentially, they have a common cellular deficiency.

Simple? Not really, but at least it was a plausible explanation and they could give me reasons why I was feeling as I was.

By late July 1995, I knew much more about my illness, and was getting some help that was actually working. I was feeling better — and so was the team. We had come from 45 points down at three-quarter time to beat Hawthorn at the Gabba. It was the biggest final-quarter comeback for a win in AFL history and set the Bears, 14th on the ladder going into that game, on a remarkable surge to the finals. It was the turning point in the club's brief history. We won six of the last seven, losing only to minor premiers

Carlton, and snuck into the finals for the first time, albeit with just 10 wins from a 22-game season. About as low a pass mark as you'll get. We'd beaten Essendon and Melbourne in the first two night games at the Gabba to close out the home-and-away campaign, and on the Sunday of Round 22 we needed 12th-placed Sydney to beat 10th-placed Collingwood at the SCG. Otherwise the Magpies would jump us into eighth spot. We gathered at Kelly's Hotel, South Brisbane, not far from the Gabba, and watched on television. Tony Lockett kicked seven goals and the Swans got home by 28 points. We were in! And, though I wasn't really part of it, I was absolutely rapt for the players. They'd been through so much, and finally they were going to play in the finals.

I went to Melbourne the following week to be part of this historic occasion. I'd been doing a regular spot with 'The Coodabeen Champions' on 3AW throughout the season, and I worked as a boundary rider for the Geelong–Footscray final on the Saturday, then joined Coodabeens front man Ian Cover in speaking at the Bears' pre-game function on the Sunday. We lost by 13 points to the eventual premiers, Carlton — we were the only team that got close to the Blues in September. It was disappointing, but everyone was enormously proud of the effort. We'd come from nowhere. The signs were all positive for the following year, and I was determined to be part of it.

I'd reached a turning point, too, via a letter from Ramon Andersson, an international kayak paddler from Perth who had overcome CFS and returned to top-level training and competition. I called him after receiving a letter from him and we spoke for more than an hour. He was a real inspiration. He was back training harder than ever before in preparation for the 1996 Olympics and I found that really encouraging. I was starting to believe I could do it.

That was important. The depression which had engulfed me for so long had probably been holding back my recovery. I wondered if ever I'd be well again. Yet here was an elite athlete who had been through what I was going through and had bounced back. He made the final of the K4 1000 in Atlanta, finishing ninth, after he'd been part of a bronze medal-winning team in the same event in Barcelona in 1992. To do that you've got to believe you *can* do it and as soon as I overcame this hurdle I started to improve.

*   *   *

If Barry Sheene was the face of CFS in Australia during its infancy, I inadvertently became something similar in 1995. It wasn't anything I set out to do, but through my football profile and the media interest in my condition it was unavoidable. And just as Barry had been only too happy to help me, I was happy to try to help others.

I was overwhelmed by the letters, phone calls and faxes I received at the football club — and, as technology changed, emails. It started when I was first diagnosed with CFS and went on for years. And whenever my CFS got a re-run in the media or I wasn't able to play because of my illness they'd flood in again. There were three categories — people offering support and advice, for which I was enormously grateful, and people who were asking for my advice, while hundreds more wrote to say thank you. Always prefacing their remarks by saying that they didn't want to appear selfish, they weren't saying they were glad I was sick, but they were pleased they could now say they had what Alastair Lynch had. After months of the same frustration I'd been through, they now had someone to identify with. I wasn't offended — I knew exactly what they meant.

At first I tried to reply to every message, but it quickly became too much. One day at the club, football department secretary Nicole Duncan presented me with a big Australia Post plastic box full of letters. 'What's that?' I asked. 'Your mail,' she told me.

So, with the help of Lions communications manager Peter Blucher, I drafted a letter which expressed my gratitude and outlined what I'd done to set myself on the road to recovery. He distributed this on my behalf, often to as many as 50 people a week.

In the letter I tried to sympathise with and encourage the CFS sufferers, explaining that I understood the frustration they were going through and that there was no need for them to feel isolated. I tried to reassure them that there was hope and that they would get better, even if salvation sometimes seemed a long way off. I quoted the CFS studies at the University of Newcastle, and the blood tests which identified deficiencies in my immune system, and at least gave me a reason for my headaches, muscle pain and lack of energy.

I explained that Dr Whiting and the football club's medical and conditioning team and I had together formulated an exercise program which allowed me to train without suffering the most severe effects of CFS. The program started with very light weights and minimal exercise. I would lift 30–40 per cent of my normal capacity and slowly graduate from short walks to slow jogs. There's a fine line, which only the patient can judge. My program was to do a little but not make myself tired, and make sure I gave myself plenty of rest. I started off lifting 20kg on a bench press and walking 200 metres.

I also outlined the strict diet that I would stick to for the remainder of my playing career. The key elements were plenty of fruit and minimal simple sugars (such as chocolate), a minimum of two litres of water a day, and definitely no alcohol. Hydration was critical, and alcohol was counterproductive. Essentially, what I was trying to do was give my body and my immune system every possible resource to fight off the CFS and fix itself.

I believed then and still believe that exercise is most important. But it's difficult to identify exactly how much exercise is optimal. In my experience, CFS sufferers need to stimulate their bodies. As much as they might feel like spending all day in bed when CFS is at its peak, it doesn't do any good. They've got to do a little something, and gradually build it up. Even if it's only walking to the letterbox or to the local shops if they are close by. Patients need to listen to their body: it provides the best guide to the middle ground between enough exercise and too much. Err on the cautious side, I'd say, because it's easy to overdo it. And be patient. It's always going to take time. Over time I modified the letter we sent to CFS sufferers. As I learned something new and verified that it was helpful I'd include it in the letter.

I also used a product called Vital Edge, a comprehensive nutritional supplement which helps feed the immune system essential micro-nutrients. It was researched and developed in Australia, and released in 1995. I don't mind giving it a free plug for one simple reason — it helped me.

The most difficult part about treating CFS is the individuality of it all. There are no guarantees that what works for me will work for anyone else. And vice versa. I never really knew whether what I did as a professional sportsman had the same effect on a non-sportsman. All I could do was offer my advice and support.

As 1995 progressed, even though I'd given up any thought of playing football again that year, I was slowly starting to feel better. Still, I was always keen to talk with anyone who might be able to help, and I remember vividly a tremendous chat I had in December 1995 with West Indian cricket captain and CFS sufferer Richie Richardson. He didn't come to me — I went to him. The

Windies were in Australia for the one-day series of 1995–96 and they were using the Brisbane Bears' gymnasium and changing facilities. I said hello, and initially I got the polite, 'Yeah, how you going?' reply. He probably thought, 'Who is this pest?' But as soon as I mentioned CFS and told him who I was and that I'd had a similar problem, his mood changed completely. We sat in front of my locker for the best part of an hour and exchanged stories. I enjoyed it, and I got the feeling he did, too.

Robert Craddock, a leading Brisbane-based Australian cricket writer with the News Limited group, tells the story of how, when he and the Australian team arrived in the Windies for the four-Test series in 1995, the first thing that struck everyone was how much Richardson's physical presence had changed. It was Richardson's comeback series after almost 12 months out of Test cricket, and he would play just 10 more Test matches before retiring, aged 33, in March 1996.

'Richie Richardson was one of the really terrific people in world cricket, and it was a tragedy to see him reduced to a shadow of his former self on and off the field,' said 'Crash' Craddock. 'He lost a lot of weight, and instead of being the nuggety, muscle-bound player he was in his prime, he was quite thin and frail. Mark Taylor would go to pre-match meetings with Richie and the match officials and come away wondering if Richie was really with it. He lost a lot of confidence — no doubt it affected him physically and mentally. He was never the same again. Whether by coincidence or otherwise, the West Indies lost their first series in 15 years.'

I found Richie Richardson to be a fantastic person. We talked about the frustration we shared of having an illness which nobody could really explain or treat, and the scepticism that existed among many around us. We found many of our symptoms were similar. He told me of his total lack of energy and how he felt like he'd been hit by a truck — it could have been me saying those very same words.

Just as it was good for Roosy to see first-hand what CFS can do to people when it strikes really hard, it was good for me to have a world-class sportsman like the West Indian cricket captain to talk to. There was a real understanding between us; we tended to feed off each other and could relate to what the other was saying. It's a connection that CFS sufferers invariably have.

We shared a big problem with concentration, which is often a major symptom of CFS. I was finding it difficult to do things like drive and read, but for him it was a different thing — playing cricket for long periods in warm conditions. With a cricket ball flying at him when he was batting and fielding it was dangerous and he had to have his wits about him. Yet, even though he was back in the international arena, he admitted he still struggled at times. Nevertheless, just playing cricket helped him cope with his overall health situation.

I got the impression that Richie took something away from our conversation, which was good because he wasn't getting a lot of joy from the medical fraternity in the Caribbean. And certainly I took inspiration from his comeback. It was the Ramon Andersson experience all over again, except it was more specific to my situation. Ramon had got back into full training and was working harder than ever before, but Richie was more in my category — well enough to play at a reasonable level without being at his best. That was an important lesson. It helped me realise there was a middle ground, and that maybe, just as he had done, I'd have to accept that. Even if I would never be able to work hard enough to get fit enough to get back to what I was in 1993, I might have to be satisfied with simply being able to compete in the sport I loved.

It was amazing how many other leading Australian sportsmen have suffered from CFS, and as the months progressed I often found myself treated as an 'expert' and giving advice, just as Richie Richardson, Ramon Andersson and Barry Sheene had done for me. I spoke at length with Olympic swimmer Linley Frame, who was flattened by CFS after she'd won a world breaststroke championship. She came to Brisbane as a sports commentator and we got together for coffee at Park Road, Milton. All I could do was give her the benefit of my experience and reassure her, just as others had done for me, that you could get over it and get back into top-level competition.

Linda Halfweeg was another who came to me for help. She was a teenage prodigy who had reached the top as an ironwoman only to crash heavily. I spoke to her several times on the phone without meeting her, and it was great to see her get back into competition. I met her in 2004 when she was doing some work experience with Channel Seven.

One of the things that struck me after talking to people like Linley and Linda was how hard it would be to be playing an individual sport and have CFS. I always had my teammates to lean on, and they were fantastic. I was able to compromise a little and, without getting back to peak fitness, at least get to a level where I could make a worthwhile contribution. I never got back to my fitness levels of 1993–94, because, as the lessons of 1999 would teach me, I knew not to push the boundaries too far. But in a team sport that was acceptable. In an individual sport like swimming or surf lifesaving you could never do that, because you compete against yourself as much as you compete against others. There would always be that desire to keep pushing the limit. I don't know whether I would ever have made it back to top-level competition had I been in that sort of situation.

Any number of top-level sportsmen and women have suffered from CFS. People like surfer Layne Beachley, Olympic kayak gold medallist Clint Robinson, marathon swimmer Shelley Taylor-Smith, Test cricketers Simon Katich and Matthew Nicholson, tennis player Evie Dominikovic, sprinter Sharon Cripps, triathlete Craig Walton, swimmer Duncan Armstrong, ex-swimmer turned television personality Johanna Griggs, and Tracey Menzies, coach of swimming megastar Ian Thorpe. And Krishna Stanton, the former wife of Lions physiotherapist Peter Stanton, who recovered not just from CFS but also from stress fractures to win a silver medal in the 2002

Commonwealth Games marathon. In AFL circles, my former teammate Troy Lehmann displayed CFS-type symptoms, as did Richmond's former No. 1 draft pick Anthony Banik and Kris Massie, formerly of Carlton and now at Adelaide. It has also affected the Duchess of Kent, international entertainers Cher and Sinead O'Connor, playwright Sir Andrew Lloyd Webber, and Australian actor/celebrity Tottie Goldsmith.

I could go on and on. These are just people I'm aware of after research for this book. What does it tell you? There is no rhyme or reason about the type of person who contracts CFS. No real pattern. But for every so-called celebrity who has CFS there are hundreds of people without a public profile. Like Honey Bacon, wife of former Tasmanian Premier Jim Bacon, Christine Oakley, wife of long-time AFL boss Ross Oakley, Donna Johnson, wife of Western Bulldogs footballer Brad Johnson, and Karin Kemp, wife of former West Coast footballer Dean Kemp. It knows no limits and boundaries.

Sadly, Jim Bacon died in 2004, leaving Honey to continue her fight against CFS on her own. Christine Oakley was forced to resign her position as headmistress of the junior school of Wesley College in Melbourne in 1993. She says she's now 70–75 per cent recovered, but is still cautious not to overdo things. Karin Kemp, once an international model, had five bad years with CFS and 10 years overall but she's now quite well. And Donna Johnson, forced to take 12 months off work at the worst of her illness and now a stay-at-home mother, still has her ups and downs, but has learned to cope. As you do.

Over the years I've spoken at quite a few seminars and meetings related to CFS, and I find them really mixed occasions. It's terribly sad to see so many people affected by a condition which I wouldn't wish on my worst enemy, but it's pleasing to think I might be able to offer a little help.

Another CFS patient I met is Leanne McKnoulty, who says she developed CFS in the early 1990s after repeated chemical exposure while working in X-ray departments, repeated chest infections skiing in Austria and a one-off incident in which she was bitten by a tick.

I didn't know it at the time, but I met her at a CFS talk at the Novotel Hotel in Brisbane in 1998. She arrived late and took the only seat left, which just happened to be next to me in the front row. She had no idea who Alastair Lynch was; she had come to the seminar out of sheer desperation.

It's a story that typifies what CFS is like, and it is worth repeating. Leanne told me she hadn't wanted to admit she had CFS until she saw hundreds of people in the same room with the same condition and realised that living in denial was worse than living with it and trying to get help. With the help of several different medical practitioners, Dr Whiting among them, she's well enough now to lead a reasonably normal life providing she looks after herself.

That is exactly the message for CFS sufferers: there is nothing to be ashamed of about having CFS, and there is an answer. It might take time, but with patience and persistence you can get on top of it.

Leanne is so committed to the cause that after hearing I was writing a book about my fight with CFS, she volunteered to do some of the research. Thanks.

The most pleasing thing is that now CFS is a recognised condition. It is acknowledged by the World Health Organization. People don't screw up their face and shake their head at the mention of what was once so wrongly and inconsiderately termed 'yuppie flu'. There is no disputing that CFS is different from anxiety and depression; for a long time they were thought to be the same thing. We've come a long way, and that in itself is a big plus for CFS sufferers.

Each year CFS sufferers worldwide recognise International CFS Awareness Day — 12 May. This is the

birthday of Florence Nightingale, who is known as the
founder of modern nursing and pioneer of the Red Cross
movement. She apparently spent the last 50 of her 90
years pretty much bedridden with an illness similar to
what is now called CFS or ME.

But it's no celebration. Far from it. The illness is still
widely misunderstood. It is much, much more than just
chronic fatigue. Extreme exhaustion, as the name implies,
is there, but that is only part of the condition. And it is
not something that can be alleviated by prolonged rest
alone. It is a condition which extends its reach much
further.

However, mental and physical fatigue or exhaustion is
a primary symptom of CFS. It is the most common
symptom, affecting 95 per cent of CFS sufferers. And it
worsens after mental and physical exertion, often up to 24
hours later.

Also, in what to the uninitiated will seem like a total
contradiction, CFS sufferers will at times experience
dysfunctional sleep. They will find it difficult to get to
sleep, will go through long periods of broken sleep and,
even after a full night's sleep, will sometimes wake and not
feel refreshed, because they have had poor-quality sleep.
Often they will feel light-headed and dizzy.

Most CFS patients also suffer various but extreme pains. There may be a burning, aching or shooting pain in muscles and/or joints, severe headaches, or widespread tenderness. And there may be cognitive problems — a 'foggy' brain that causes problems with simple thought processes, as well as speaking, reading, writing, mathematics, short-term memory and concentration.

Less common symptoms include palpitations, muscle twitching, sensitivity to light, touch and sound, nausea, sore throat, gastrointestinal and urinary problems, tender lymph nodes, sweating and fever, intolerance to temperature changes, cold extremities, new sensitivities to foods, medications and/or chemicals, marked change in weight and a worsening of symptoms with stressors (a new infection, travel or anaesthetic, for example).

Perhaps this is why it is so widely questioned. There are too many symptoms, and the degree of CFS can vary dramatically. Most CFS patients have trouble walking long distances, climbing stairs and standing still for any length of time. They find shopping and domestic chores virtually impossible, and even simple daily tasks like showering, dressing or making a phone call can exacerbate symptoms. Patients can be mildly affected or bedridden, or anything in between.

According to Dr David S. Bell, former Harvard lecturer, staff member at Cambridge Hospital and author of *The Doctor's Guide to Chronic Fatigue Syndrome*, the confusion, controversy and misunderstandings surrounding the illness have led directly to an increased burden of suffering for those who have it. He says many illnesses, such as diabetes, cancer, anxiety and depression, can cause the symptoms of chronic fatigue, but CFS is distinct from this multitude of fatigue-causing illnesses. It is a specific and unique constellation of symptoms. So he prefers the term 'chronic fatigue/immune dysfunction syndrome' (CFIDS), because it combines the symptom of fatigue with the presence of immune-system markers, thus separating it from generic chronic fatigue.

The CFS Association of Australia advises that there are about 150,000 CFS sufferers in Australia. More people suffer from CFS than from HIV or Multiple Sclerosis. According to a 2000 report from the Royal Australasian College of Physicians, CFS costs the Australian economy $416 million a year in lost work time and is a major reason for absenteeism from school, with up to 50 per cent of children suffering from CFS missing anything from several weeks to a whole term of the school year. Some people cannot work for 12 months at a time. Yet government funding for research into CFS is minimal.

Between 65 per cent and 80 per cent of CFS sufferers develop the condition suddenly, usually after an infection or a series of infections; 30 per cent of sufferers have the illness for between 10 and 15 years, and a further 27 per cent have it for between five and ten years.

It's no surprise, then, that in the United States, the National Institute of Health, the Center for Disease Control, the Food and Drug Administration and the Social Security Administration all recognise CFS as a serious, often debilitating illness. CFS has been declared a No. 1 priority disease, along with tuberculosis and AIDS, by the Centers for Disease Control.

Yet for the uninitiated, it's still dreadfully difficult to comprehend. So what's it like? Imagine having the worst case of flu you can, add an extreme hangover and the exhaustion of a 20km run barefoot on the road, and maybe you are getting something close.

Even without exercising, I used to get a throbbing ache through my legs, as if I'd run 10km on concrete without any shock-absorbent shoes. The Queensland Academy of Sport tested me often, and found that my resting lactic acid levels were equivalent to those of Simon Black, Lions teammate and Brownlow medallist, in the middle of a peak training session.

And the physical symptoms are only part of it. The psychological drain, caused partly by the uncertainty of CFS and partly by the stigma attached to this supposedly undefined illness, is a huge part of it, too.

I've had plenty of 'magic potions' shown to me; I'm sure they work for some people but not for others. All you can do is make your own decisions, based on your own expert advice, and persevere with what works for you.

It's imperative, too, that the people near and dear to CFS sufferers offer unwavering support. I was fortunate to have a wonderful network of family and friends, and a football club that was equally supportive. But most important was my ever-loving wife, without whom I would have given up the fight long ago.

On 1 October 1995 Peta and I were married at St Mark's Church in Camberwell, Melbourne. John Blakey was best man and Paul Roos, my brother Manuel and Peter Berne, a long-time close mate from my primary school days, were groomsmen. My other brother, Vaughan, was at sea with work and couldn't get time off. Even his wife Jodie couldn't come because she had to look after their children. The reception at Rippon Lea Estate,

Elsternwick, was a fantastic occasion. I didn't have a drink. Not then. And not during our 10-day honeymoon on Turtle Island, Fiji, where everything was laid on in lavish style. I wasn't about to jeopardise the upward trend in my health. A week later, after a short stay with Ross Lyon and his then girlfriend, now wife, Kirsten, Peta and I moved into our new home at Chapel Hill. We'd built it on what was just a block of dirt at the start, but I hadn't been much help. Most times the builders arrived to discuss the plans or construction I was stuck in bed or struggling with headaches. Now I was beginning to look forwards.

7

MY FAVOURITE MERGER

I'm no historian, but I do know that 4 July is American Independence Day. To me, however, it's a date whose importance is not so much separation and independence but union and dependence. A merger. For on 4 July 1996 my old football club joined with my new club to become the force with which I would enjoy my greatest football moments.

It was a normal Thursday at the Gabba. The Brisbane Bears were preparing for their Round 14 visit to Football Park to meet the Adelaide Crows. We were not long off the training track and were enjoying our customary pasta meal when word filtered through from the south that the Bears had merged with Fitzroy.

Peter Blucher, our communications manager, had received a phone call from CEO Andrew Ireland in Melbourne. 'Get ready — all hell is about to break loose,' he told him. And it did. Suddenly, even if only temporarily, the focus switched from the present to the future and a historic football moment.

It had been one of the all-time coups. As the only Brisbane player with a Fitzroy background I finished pictured on the front page of the paper in my old Lions jumper, which I had stored in a cupboard at home.

The merger happened so quickly it was incredible. All the speculation had been that cash-strapped Fitzroy would merge with North Melbourne. The Kangaroos had made a massive play for the Lions and, like most people, I expected it to go ahead.

Fitzroy had struggled to meet the ever-escalating costs of AFL football for the better part of a decade. Several times they'd been miraculously saved at the 11th hour. In 1986 Fitzroy-based investment company Hecron came to the rescue. In 1993 local trucking millionaire Bernie Ahern lent the club $750,000 to keep the doors open. And in late 1994 the Nauru Insurance Corporation had come to the party with what was basically a $1.25 million loan. Ironically, it was the Nauruans who forced the club to finally admit defeat in their fight for solvency. On 28 June the Nauru Insurance Corporation appointed an administrator in an effort to recoup the money Fitzroy owed to them, effectively taking the matter out of the club's hands and making a merger inevitable. The only question was who they would join with. Fitzroy president Dyson Hore-Lacy was strongly in favour of the North Melbourne union, but the Roos were trumped by some clever backroom manoeuvring by the Bears contingent. Six days after the administrator took over the deal was done.

I'd followed Fitzroy's fortunes closely since moving to Brisbane. If you've been at Fitzroy, a part of the club stays with you, as I've said already. There was such a strong personal connection that it was impossible for me to separate myself from the club entirely. I cared about the people. And the wonderful history, tradition and spirit of Fitzroy, which dated back beyond the formation of the then Victorian Football League to 1884.

I hadn't given the proposed Fitzroy–North Melbourne merger a lot of thought. It seemed a formality. If a merger was the only alternative to extinction for Fitzroy, then it was a good alternative. Better to share an existence than have no existence at all.

In hindsight, I feel the Brisbane–Fitzroy merger was much the better deal. It brought together a proud old club with a wonderful history and an emerging new force in a rapidly expanding football market. A perfect fit.

The Brisbane merger offered Fitzroy a genuine lifeline. The name, the colours and the club song would live on. Forever. Sure, the team would be based in Brisbane and things wouldn't be quite the same, but things weren't going to be the same anyway. At least Brisbane didn't have a long and proud history of its own to protect and foster. The Brisbane Lions was definitely the best way for all parties to go. And through time a genuine bond between the two groups developed. A dependence on one another for shared success.

It was a really emotional time for all concerned. I was happy because I had a stake in both clubs, but for others it wasn't so cut and dried. Not at all. It was sad that Fitzroy had ceased to exist in their own right, but at least they would still have a genuine presence on the national football scene. And for Brisbane there were some significant benefits.

Short-term, Brisbane inherited eight Fitzroy players and what was left of the $6 million merger incentive package offered by the AFL after Fitzroy's debts were paid.

It was about $1.2 million. Not a lot of money in big picture terms, but nothing to sneeze at.

Most importantly, though, the merger created something that Brisbane were always going to struggle to establish: a strong and vibrant supporter base in Melbourne. At first, the support among Fitzroy people for the Brisbane Lions was limited. Not everyone came across. Some, understandably, went with North Melbourne. Some followed other clubs. And some just faded out of football. But as the club's success grew and we started winning premierships, the number of supporters grew. One of the really special times for me was sharing this success with lifetime Lions/Fitzroy fans who hadn't won a flag since 1944.

It says a lot about the passion that football generates that people's lives can be so affected by what happens to their club. A lot of Fitzroy people were genuinely shattered by the merger. They felt their club had been taken away; I understood that. They couldn't go and watch their team train during the week. And we would only play in Melbourne six or seven times a year. It was different and difficult. All the Brisbane Lions could do was be true to their pre-merger commitment to uphold Fitzroy's history and tradition. There were three components which provided a massive start — the name Lions, the jumper, which was predominantly the Fitzroy strip with a lion instead of the FFC (Fitzroy Football Club) monogram, and the club song, sung to the tune of the French National Anthem, as the Fitzroy song had been. Thereafter, people had to make up their own mind.

The Brisbane players were divided on the merger. I was in the minority. Many of the others were largely neutral. Football was a job for them. Their passion lay with their teammates, and their concerns lay with the present and the future. The past wasn't a big consideration.

But for players who had been with the Bears for a long time it was a very real issue. Michael Voss was at first really disappointed. Like fellow teammates Marcus Ashcroft, Shaun Hart, Darryl White, Richard Champion and Matthew Kennedy, he'd been with Brisbane since the dark old days at Carrara, when they'd been known as the Bad News Bears. He'd experienced the times when nobody wanted to know the club. When they were an embarrassment. And now, at last, the Bears jumper had started to mean something. We'd played in the finals in 1995 and were going along nicely in 1996. For Vossy, to lose the Bears identity which he and others had fought so long and so hard to establish was a big thing.

In time Vossy and others would soften. They'd see the wisdom in the merger, and the benefits. Their passion for the Brisbane Lions would become so strong that the Bears era would be confined to the history books. Never forgotten, because it's so important to remember where you've come from, but replaced with a passion just as strong for the club that was going to take them all the way to the top.

At the time of the merger there were still nine rounds of football, plus finals, to be played in 1996. There was a premiership to be won. And the Bears, under new coach John Northey, were right in the picture. We sat sixth on the ladder, with eight wins and a draw from 13 games, after fluctuating between first and third for the first 12 weeks. Me? I was just happy to be playing again, after having missed virtually the entire 1995 season.

Some not so attentive observers might have thought the club had recruited a new player to wear jumper No. 11 — he was much heavier and a different shape from the player who had last worn No. 11 for the Bears, in Round 1, 1995. Instead of a fit 98kg, as I'd been at my peak, I was a tubby 108kg. And the extra weight was all fat. It wasn't something I was comfortable with, but it was something I had to learn to live with. Because the only other option was not playing at all. I couldn't train enough to do anything about it.

I'd not been able to do a lot of training over the summer of 1995–96, but I had done enough to at least be able to play. I didn't do much on the track, especially when it was hot, but I was able to do some work in the gym providing I gave myself sufficient rest time in between. I also did minimal work on the bike and in the pool.

Coach Northey was very good to me. He was new to the club and would have been frustrated, like Robert Walls before him, that I wasn't able to contribute like the other players. But not once did he make me feel like that. He accepted the situation and made the most of it. Taking that stance is very important for anyone who is involved with CFS sufferers.

There was one thing I had to get my mind around — that my days of playing as a running centre half forward were over. I simply didn't have the aerobic capacity any more. That disappointed me, because in my prime I had loved the challenge of really taking on an opponent athletically. Now I was a stay-at-home full forward.

And opposition teams were getting smarter. They knew my physical limitations, so my opponent would try to run off me at every opportunity. I couldn't chase, so it virtually created a loose man. That's where my teammates were so good. They were mindful of the situation and were always alert to try to help out, and to pick up my opponent if he was in a dangerous position and looked like getting the ball.

The other players were fantastic at training, too. I didn't do an awful lot on the track with them, but when I did they were always keen to help out. If I was struggling after a drill, not quite ready to go again, they'd push up through the line and give me that extra 30 seconds which would make the difference. I wasn't doing what everyone else was expected to do, which went against everything a sporting team is built on, but they never made me feel I wasn't part of it. For that I will always be grateful.

My first game back in 1996 was unforgettable. Especially my first goal. It was Round 1, against Footscray at the Gabba. Trent Bartlett kicked it in from the wing and I led out in front of what was once the Cricketers Club to take a mark. When I slotted it from outside 50m the roar was fantastic. Anyone who says spectators don't make a difference is kidding themselves. That was one special moment in my career and gave me just the tonic I needed at just the right time.

We had an interesting goal-square pairing in 1996, and managed to be quite effective. There was a fat bloke on the comeback trail and the oldest bloke in the League, who was in the twilight of his career. Roger Merrett had been an icon for the club. Having moved from Essendon to the Bears in 1988, he'd been the face of AFL football in Queensland. And a fantastic player and captain. But by April 1996 he was 36 and unable to play 120 minutes a week. So it worked out nicely. We often operated in tandem off the interchange bench; when one needed a spell the other could take over.

Together, the old bloke and the bloke who seemed like he was old managed to kick 74 goals in 1996 and help put the Bears right in the finals picture. For four weeks early in the season and again after Round 21 we sat on top of the ladder. Going into Round 22 we only had to beat 11th-placed Collingwood at Victoria Park to secure the minor premiership. It was something Brisbane had never done. They'd never even got close. Their best previous finish was eighth, in 1995.

We blew it. And in hindsight we blew a golden opportunity to win a premiership. Against an under-manned Magpie outfit which lost key players Sav Rocca and Damien Monkhorst on the morning of the game, we lost by 49 points. Instead of first, we finished third. And instead of the easier passage through the finals, we were going to have to do it the hard way. Who knows what might have happened if we'd beaten Collingwood? It makes you realise yet again that you've got to play for the moment, because you never know what the future will bring. We were fortunate that our time would come, but it might have been otherwise. This might have been our one and only opportunity at football glory.

As it turned out, we beat Essendon by a point in the first Gabba final, smashed Carlton by 97 points at the Gabba the following week and then, after a heavy injury toll, lost to eventual premiers North Melbourne by 36 points at the MCG in the preliminary final.

If we'd beaten Collingwood in Round 22 it would have meant a different opponent in the first week of the finals, a week off if we'd won, and then a home preliminary final against some team other than North. We might well have played in the grand final. We might even have won. A lesson learned.

The qualifying final against Essendon was my 150th game and my finals debut. Finals football is the reason you play. It's the big stage that every player aspires to play on. It had been a long wait, and after missing 1995 it was a huge bonus. Grand finals aside, it was probably the most memorable game of my career. Essendon's Gavin Wanganeen hit the post from close range in the last minute, after the Bombers had clawed their way back from a 27 point deficit early in the fourth quarter. It was one of those games that sticks in your mind, not just because of my personal milestone, but because of the barnstorming Bombers comeback — which could so easily have got them over the line.

It was terribly disappointing to finish within one game of the grand final, but personally, 52 goals in 18 matches, including 13 goals in the three finals and seven against Carlton in the semi-final, was a big confidence booster. I was still exhausted after a game and would take two or three days to recover, but at least I was on an upward path. I always knew it was going to be a long, slow process, and that I couldn't afford to rush it. I had to be patient.

If I needed a reminder, it came in the qualifying final against Essendon. I was in the play a lot early and had four marks inside 10 minutes. I kicked two goals and two out of bounds. The adrenaline was pumping. After such a long wait to play in September I wasn't going to waste it. I'd even chased my opponent down the ground a couple of times.

But five minutes later I was off the ground. Spent. I was on and off the bench for the rest of the night.

At least, though, I'd played virtually a full season and had made a reasonable team contribution. After 1995, every game was a bonus. I was enjoying being back. And, importantly, I again felt I belonged.

The summer of 1996–97 was a busy time and an unusual one, because the club went from Bears to Lions. The official changeover happened on 1 November 1996. You've got no idea how difficult it is to get the change firmly fixed in your mind. If there had been fines for every time somebody said Bears instead of Lions we would have made a fortune. All of a sudden, too, the ton of training gear in the cupboard was redundant. We weren't allowed to wear it. It was branded Bears. So bit by bit I gave it away to schools, charities and anyone else who asked.

One day I remember vividly from this 1997 pre-season was the first Brisbane Lions Family Day in Melbourne. It was Sunday, 16 March. The first time the merged club had been on public display to the Fitzroy faithful. I wasn't sure what to expect — but I certainly didn't expect the 3500 people who turned up at Fitzroy's old Brunswick Street headquarters. It was fantastic. I spent two and a half hours signing autographs and catching up with people I hadn't seen for three years. Brad Boyd, the last Fitzroy captain, said he'd never seen a crowd like it at this sort of function. And Scott McIvor, another ex-Fitzroy boy returning to Brunswick Street, said he was embarrassed by the overwhelming response. It was sensational.

Among the crowd was a group of people special to me. The old Lynch Mob. They were back. The club magazine, *The Lion's Tale*, published a story about the Mob — or the working-class coterie, as they called themselves. It had a group of a dozen hard-core key members — the numbers jumped to 100-plus if the team was going well. Consensus suggested that Kevin Court had been the instigator of the Mob, and that the group had been formed one day at Princes Park when, coincidentally, Richard Osborne kicked 11 goals for Fitzroy against Melbourne in 1989, but it didn't matter. They even published their own newsletters — 80 in total — and had their own end-of-season trip. Apparently when I'd left at the end of 1993 there were 128 official members of the Mob.

Wayne Kelly and Scott Fletcher assumed the role of spokesmen for the Mob when *The Lion's Tale* tackled the difficult task of interviewing them. 'It [the merger] was inevitable, and we all thought Fitzroy would just fold. It's good that we've joined with a club that is in it for the right reasons rather than just the $6 million,' they said. 'We've still got the colours and the jumper, and Brisbane are willing to take on board our tradition lock, stock and barrel rather than just take us over. We couldn't wish for anything better.'

I don't imagine it would have been easy trying to interview the Mob, but the intrepid club reporter managed to catch the names of another 10. So, with apologies to those who didn't manage to register, there were Mark and Bradley Kelly, Steven and Haydn 'spelt like Bunton' Fletcher, John and Brian Zwiers, Cameron Hearn, Wade Britnell, Denis Quinn and Mark Higgins.

Season 1996 had been Roger Merrett's 19th season in the AFL and his last. He retired after the preliminary final loss to North Melbourne. And so, for the first time since 1990, the club needed a new captain. It was a dilemma. There was no automatic choice. Michael McLean, Marcus Ashcroft and I had been vice-captains under Roger but there was also a strong case for Michael Voss, who had shared the 1996 Brownlow Medal with Essendon's James Hird.

Contrary to a lot of media reports, I did not have it written into my contract that I would be captain of the club. Yes, it had been offered to me as an incentive to move north three years earlier, but that wasn't the way I wanted to receive such an honour. I wanted to earn it for the leadership I could bring to the side. Anything else would have been embarrassing.

John Northey and the brains trust opted for co-captains — Vossy and me. It was nothing new. St Kilda had shared the leadership between Nathan Burke and Stewart Loewe in 1996, and Geelong had had a real captaincy roundabout, which included Gary Ablett, Barry Stoneham and Ken Hinkley in 1995–96. It was a good, commonsense decision. Vossy was still young, only 21, and he had enough pressure on him as a Brownlow medallist. He didn't need to be over-burdened. And I was only 12 months back from a year off through illness. I didn't need it either. But together we could share the workload, especially the off-field duties. In a developing football state like Queensland, that was an important part of the role. You had to be an ambassador for the club, be available for sponsors and the media. Solo, it would have been a huge ask. But together it wasn't an unreasonable ask.

I wouldn't have accepted the job if I hadn't had a reasonable 1996. If I hadn't played pretty much all year and didn't think I could return to my best. It wouldn't have been the right thing to do for the club or me. I always knew Vossy would end up in the job. He was such a standout. I fully expected him to develop into a great captain, as he would do later, but I felt that if I could help out for a couple of years and soften his transition to full-scale leadership that would be a good thing. It was still a great honour for me. I'd been vice-captain at Fitzroy for three years and vice-captain at Brisbane for three years, including the year I didn't play. To have the joint captaincy was a huge thing.

It was an altogether new-look leadership team. Marcus Ashcroft and Craig Lambert were appointed vice-captains, and Matthew Clarke and Richard Champion were deputy vice-captains. If the club made one mistake it was to exclude Brad Boyd, who had headed the group of eight Fitzroy players chosen under the merger guidelines. They said at the time that it was to lessen the burden on the ex-Fitzroy captain but I think it was a bit of a slap in the face. Boydo didn't say anything; he wouldn't. That wasn't his go. But after doing such a sensational job under such difficult circumstances at Fitzroy in the two years before the merger, he deserved a leadership role.

As it turned out, it didn't really matter. The career of this champion was cut short by chronic back problems.

He'd play only 15 games in three years in Brisbane Lions colours before being forced into retirement at the end of the 1999 season. One of those games was as good as you'll see. It was Leigh Matthews' first match at the helm for Brisbane: Round 1, 1999, against St Kilda at the Gabba. Boydo had 29 possessions and kicked four goals as acting captain. We really didn't see enough of this tall, loping midfielder who had a great ability to find the football.

Boydo and Simon Hawking, who would never play at senior level for the Brisbane Lions, were the only two ex-Fitzroy players I'd played with in Melbourne. John Barker was at the club in 1993 but he didn't play in the seniors. And Chris Johnson, Jarrod Molloy, Scott Bamford, Nick Carter and Shane Clayton were post-1993 signings.

The merger was a delicate issue because it unsettled the psyche of the playing group and the club as a whole. There was nothing intentional or sinister in this. The Fitzroy boys certainly weren't ostracised. There was no 'us v them' mentality. Everyone did their utmost to make them feel part of things, but it was inevitable that with such a significant change there would be disruption. And there was. At the end of 1996 the Brisbane players knew exactly where they sat in the pecking order. Then overnight, eight newcomers who had a higher status than normal first-year draftees were dropped into the group.

The worst thing that could have happened was the massive and immediate expectation built up in the media. After the Brisbane Lions beat Essendon 15.13 (103) to 8.7 (55) in the first round of the Ansett Cup in 1997, Kevin Sheedy started talking about a superclub. About who would play Brisbane in the grand final. You could see where he was coming from. After all, the Bears had finished third in 1996 and had been strengthened by the inclusion of eight Fitzroy players. The Bombers boss, one of the great coaching marketers in the game's history and never one to miss an opportunity, quickly helped build a pressure that we didn't need.

It was never going to be as simple as that. Irrespective of how much talent a team has, the people in it must work together. Otherwise, the results just don't happen. We were always going to take time to blend. And we did.

In 1997 we started 2–6, then went 7–1 to be 9–7 and fifth on the ladder after 16 rounds. We were still fifth a fortnight on, but we didn't win another game. We fell into the finals despite three losses and a draw from our last four games, and were eliminated in week 1 of the finals by minor premiers St Kilda, who subsequently lost the grand final to Adelaide.

*   *   *

About a third of the way through the year I had a change of role, reverting to my former position at fullback. I got through the year all right without doing a lot on the track. I was still taking time to recover after games. Often Sunday, Monday and even Tuesday were spent pretty much in bed — you wouldn't see much of me until Wednesday each week. But relatively speaking, my health was much better.

We had deliberately held off having children while I was sick. I wanted to be well enough to enjoy them and to be able to offer Peta some decent help. It wasn't something we could contemplate while I was bed-ridden for extended periods. We never discussed exactly how many children we wanted but it was always two and maybe three.

I'd played a full season of football in 1996 and while I was still a bit up and down we figured I was well enough to start a family. And the birth of our first child, our daughter Madison, in September 1997, was the perfect tonic to help boost me along a little bit more.

I've got to admit I didn't know much about kids until I had one of my own and all of a sudden I understand what people mean when they say 'it's different when it's your own'. It really is. She gave me another purpose in life, something outside football to focus on and keep things in perspective a little. I didn't just want to get back to full health to play football — I had a family to provide for and to enjoy everyday things with.

I remember when Madison was about 18 months old I copped a bit of a spray from the coach after an ordinary game early in 1999 and when I got home and opened the door feeling a bit downcast I heard her little footsteps running towards me. She didn't care whether I'd played well or played badly. A few years on, when she was old enough to understand, she asked me how many goals I'd kicked after another pretty average day. I told her I'd only kicked one goal and she replied, 'It doesn't matter Dad.' She was right — it didn't matter. Not really.

I've heard a lot of guys say they desperately wanted a boy when they were contemplating a family but I was never like that — especially after Madison was born. I'm not really a cuddly sort of person but I loved having a little girl to hug and kiss so much that I would have been just as happy to have another girl.

Still, when Tom followed in May 2000 I was happy because it meant Pete and I would experience both sides of the parenting situation. I'm sure I'll look forward to having a kick with him in the backyard if he's interested in footy, but right now it doesn't happen too often. He's five, and he'd rather play basketball or tennis, ride his bike, play in the cubby house or go sliding down the hill. Often he'll put on his overalls and give me a hand in the garden.

Claudia was born in July 2003 and completed our family. Another beautiful little girl. We consider ourselves so fortunate to have three happy, healthy children to whom we can devote our love and attention.

Going into 1998, expectations were high again. We felt we'd put the impact of the merger behind us and we certainly had the talent. Maybe this would be the year where we'd build on our preliminary final appearance of 1996. How wrong we would be!

Instead we went from one disaster to another. It was a classic example of how not to run a football club. Or a business. Or anything, for that matter. We were a divided group. We'd had Coopers & Lybrand in to conduct an internal survey on the football operations of the club but it didn't have the desired result. All it did was give people a licence to criticise others and push their own barrow. We had factions and personal agendas everywhere. It quickly became about survival, and coach John Northey didn't survive.

'Swoop' was a victim of all sorts of things. Many of these were beyond his control, but primarily he fell because of the poor performance of the team. We let him down. After 11 rounds we were at the bottom of the ladder, with just two wins. A 71 point hiding at the hands of Fremantle in Perth, in which Michael Voss suffered a season-ending broken leg, was the final straw. The coach was sacked four days later.

The players knew Northey was under pressure because it was all we ever read about in the papers. But I didn't know what had happened until I pulled up in the carpark for training on Wednesday, 10 June. There were TV cameras everywhere. Only when I was asked for a reaction did I know he was gone. That night Trent Bartlett and I joined a few members of the administration at Northey's house. I even allowed myself one beer. It just seemed like the right way to say thank you to a bloke who had always done the right thing by me and had patiently helped me get back into League football after he'd arrived at the club to find me asleep more often than I was awake.

On principle, I don't agree with sacking a coach mid-season. I believe that once you make a commitment you

honour that commitment. But in this case I almost think it
was the best thing. The club had fragmented dreadfully and
the coach wasn't getting the support he was entitled to
expect. There was nothing more he could have done. He'd
aged 10 years in 10 weeks, and if he'd had any hair left he
would have pulled it out. There was nowhere to turn. I really
felt for him. He was a great football man, a premiership
player at Richmond and a successful coach at Sydney,
Melbourne and the Tigers before joining Brisbane. The
strain was taking a massive toll on him — when he left, he
would at least be able to start living again. But it was a sad
way for his 22-year association with AFL football to end.

Roger Merrett, assistant coach since late in 1995, was
appointed caretaker coach for the remainder of the season.
He was keen to retain the job for the following year — he
had virtually an 11-week audition. He started with a draw
against Port Adelaide at the Gabba and wins over
Geelong away and Collingwood at home. It was typical of
what so often happens after a change of coach. Somehow,
from somewhere, people find something extra. Then the
wheels fell off again. We lost six in a row, and only a one-
point win over St Kilda in Round 22 provided any solace.

The club had become very political in the second half
of the year. There were lobby groups working all over the

place but somehow — I don't quite know how — I managed to stay out of them. There were player meetings initiated by club director Alastair Bayles, with the apparent intention of generating support for the caretaker coach to continue in 1999. I wasn't invited to attend, so when I was asked about the secret meetings on radio one day I could honestly say I didn't know what was going on.

There's nothing worse than a football club in turmoil. After Vossy's terrible injury I was left to skipper the side until I, too, went down. A Round 15 hamstring injury against West Coast, chasing a lightning fast Fraser Gehrig on a lead, did the job. I missed the next five weeks.

It had already been a difficult year. In the week of the premiership opener I had learned I had a stress fracture in my lower back. I had a choice: three months on the sideline or try to play with it. I took the latter, but it had been a bit of a struggle.

When Vossy was sidelined I felt a responsibility to try to play, even though I knew I wasn't quite right. I wanted to help us salvage something from the ruins. On the Thursday night before the Round 21 game against Richmond at the MCG I got through training at three-quarter pace and made myself available. Bad move.

You know you're not going well when you can't push through the banner. I led the team out against the Tigers and my hammie twinged again. It was a windy day, so maybe the cheer squad put some extra tape on the banner. Whatever, it was too much for me. I hobbled along for 60m or so and we ran straight into the Richmond players as they emerged through their banner. Instantly, I learned a new word: melee. It wasn't premeditated and nothing serious happened, but there was a bit of pushing and shoving. I was deemed to be one of the primary instigators because I was at the front of the group. I was fined $4000. It was a miserable end to a miserable year.

The back stress fracture and the hamstring aside, my health in 1998 had been much the same as it was in 1997. I took two or three days to recover after a game and didn't do a lot of training, but I was able to get through and make a contribution. And that despite a personally exhausting tribunal saga in May that dragged on for almost three weeks. In fact, personally there was one thing to be happy about. Although I played only 15 of 22 games and three times was off the ground with back-related hamstring problems, I was second in the best and fairest behind runaway winner Chris Scott going into Round 22. I was eventually overtaken, and finished fifth. Missing the last eight games, more or less, finally caught up with me.

So we ended season 1998 in total disarray. For the one and only time in my career, I finished with the wooden spoon. We'd been close a few times at Fitzroy but had always managed to find an escape hatch. Not this year. At least we knew we could start afresh in 1999. And little did we know that even before the Round 22 game against St Kilda — which, incidentally, sent Andrew Bews into retirement — the key element of the club's recovery program was already in place.

8

D H E A SPELLS TROUBLE

One day in late February 1998 I walked into a Brisbane health food shop. It was something I'd done dozens of times. I lived on supplements to help combat my CFS. But this was to be an altogether different day: the beginning of one of the toughest periods of my life.

Almost as a throwaway line, the bloke behind the counter said to me: 'Did you know DHEA has been added to the banned list?' No, I didn't know.

DHEA, or dehydroepiandrosterone, was something I'd been prescribed by Dr John Whiting as part of my CFS medication protocol. And the banned list the man in the shop was referring to was the International Olympic

Committee's list of substances which professional athletes were prohibited from taking. This list was the cornerstone of the AFL's Anti-Doping Code.

I immediately rang a local representative of the Australian Sports Drug Agency (ASDA). He had presented the annual anti-doping lecture to the Brisbane players several times, and had become something of a friend because his wife was a CFS sufferer. I asked what I should do and he told me there was provision for athletes to be given special permission to take banned substances if it was for legitimate medical reasons. He advised me to make an application to the AFL.

The next call I made was to Scott Clayton, Lions director of football. I told him briefly what had happened, then headed straight to the club to discuss it in detail. He said he'd make a few enquiries and then make an appointment to see Ian Collins, the AFL's General Manager — Football Operations.

I left the club, not too worried. There was a process in place and plenty of precedents — several sportspeople had been given special dispensations. I knew this because I was one of them. I'd been given permission about two years earlier to take fludrocortisone, a medication used to control severe orthostatic and postural hypertension. This too had been prescribed by Dr Whiting. Worst case, they would deny me permission to use DHEA and I'd have to find another way to cope with my CFS.

I'd begun taking both DHEA and fludrocortisone in February/March 1996 when I'd been sick for about 18 months. Under Dr Whiting's strict regime I had been having blood tests twice a week, to monitor the levels of various substances in my body and determine how best to remedy any deficiencies.

Scott Clayton met Ian Collins in Melbourne on 13 March, the day before the Lions' Ansett Cup semi-final against North Melbourne at Waverley. He tabled two letters — one from ASDA representative Tim Burke and another from Dr Whiting. Burke's letter, dated 2 March, confirmed the advice from Dr Whiting that my use of DHEA was for therapeutic purposes only and that there was provision within the AFL rules for discretionary permission to be given to allow me to continue taking it. Dr Whiting's letter, dated 11 March, detailed the history of my CFS. He wrote:

When I reviewed Alastair first he was unable to stand for even five minutes without fainting or collapsing. Since that time we have made great progress in his well-being but his condition still persists, albeit under control, and he needs constant supervision. He is on medications that I consider are essential for controlling not only his well-being on the football field but in general as well. I am confident that without them Alastair would relapse to his former state . . . Amongst the medications that he is on is the substance known as DHEA. DHEA has been one of the most important therapeutic interventions that I have come across in recent times and many of my patients would be unable to function without it. However, because of its androgenic status, it is considered to be a banned drug by both the TGA (Therapeutic Goods Authority) and the AFL. Part of my normal practice is careful monitoring of a large battery of different biochemical variables, including DHEA levels. Both Alastair and myself have been very conscious of anything that would be viewed as abuse of DHEA, and we have been very careful to avoid levels that would be considered excessive. Indeed, DHEA used in doses that put him above the normal range for his age seemed to have a negative effect on his well-being and consequently he is on a low dose that I would often even prescribe to a woman. Furthermore, his testosterone levels have never been in a range that would be considered even in the high/normal.

It didn't take long for the impact of all this to trickle down. On 16 March and 6 April I was drug-tested: once at the club, and once they knocked on the door at home. I had nothing to hide so I happily went along with the tests.

On 17 March Collins wrote to Dr Whiting acknowledging receipt of his earlier letter and seeking clarification and further detail about my treatment.

On 2 April Dr Whiting wrote back to Collins confirming that I was also taking desipramine, to help combat my sleep disorder, and fludrocortisone. He told Collins he'd treated more than 1500 CFS patients over 10 years:

The treatment protocol that I have developed has been successful in a large number of my patients in terms of symptomatic improvements. The condition, as you know, is now well recognised as being a legitimate one, with potentially serious consequences, including death from cardiac problems in the worst cases. CFS is certainly not 'all in the mind', contrary to contentions in the media and elsewhere.

I have been using DHEA as part of this protocol for approximately three years. Its beneficial effects in my patients have been profound and this medication perhaps represents one of the most significant advances in treatment that I have made over the years. The main benefits are in terms of improved sleep, improvements in cognition, improvements in muscle pains, improvements in joint integrity and in the prevention of osteo-arthritic complications of this condition.

The intention when I prescribed DHEA to player Lynch was certainly not for anabolic reasons. The fears that DHEA might have anabolic effects I believe are largely unwarranted, and in the large number of patients that I have prescribed this agent for there is not a single example of testosterone levels rising outside of the normal physiological range. Player Lynch's testosterone levels have always remained in the deficiency or low/normal range, even while on DHEA at his current dose of 50mg daily. His current urine testing by the anti-doping laboratory shows that he does not have elevated levels of epitestosterone, consistent with my contention above. Excessive anabolic hormones would certainly have resulted in a positive test. I am therefore adamant and confident that player Lynch's treatment has been entirely for therapeutic purposes.

Furthermore, I am very confident that if player Lynch's treatment was withdrawn he would relapse to his previous poor state of health. A consequence of this kind could be quite disastrous for him both physically and psychologically. Indeed, some patients' illnesses can progress, and I believe that were it not for his current therapy he would be running the risk of a progressive illness. In summary, I DO NOT consider DHEA to have anabolic properties. It is a steroid (as is cholesterol, for example) but is NOT an anabolic steroid. Furthermore, it is a naturally occurring substance derived from yams.

On 14 April 1998, as the DHEA case moved along, Dr Alan Mackenzie, the Lions club doctor, wrote to Professor Ken Hardy, the AFL Medical Commissioner, seeking permission for me to continue to take DHEA for therapeutic purposes under clause 7 of the AFL's Anti-Doping Code.

In his letter, Dr Mackenzie referred to Dr Whiting's supporting evidence and wrote:

It is his [Dr Whiting's] contention that Alastair would experience significant health impairment if the substance was withheld and that he would not be denied DHEA if he were not competing in the AFL. In view of the specialist advice, the complexity of adequately treating Chronic Fatigue Syndrome and the two negative ASDA urine tests, I feel that this application for the therapeutic use of DHEA for treatment of Chronic Fatigue Syndrome for Alastair Lynch should be given favourable consideration.

On 15 April 1998 Ian Collins came to Brisbane. I met him with Scott Clayton and Lions CEO Andrew Ireland in the Lions boardroom. I walked Collins through the whole story. How I'd become ill in September 1994. How I'd missed virtually the entire 1995 season. How I'd battled to find any answers until Dr Jack Kennedy at least diagnosed the condition. How I'd tried any number of treatments until Dr Whiting had managed to at least help get me back on track, and back playing football. And how he'd prescribed DHEA. As he'd done for many of his CFS patients.

On 17 April Dr Peter Harcourt, the AFL's Deputy Medical Commissioner, wrote to Dr Mackenzie denying my request for permission to keep taking DHEA. Dr

Harcourt claimed in the letter that while the AFL's Anti-Doping Code did allow for the use of prohibited substances under certain circumstances, it stated that anabolic steroids could not be permitted. He claimed the DHEA was an anabolic steroid and so denied permission.

This opened a real can of worms about the definition of DHEA. It was a substance that was readily available over the counter in health food stores and pharmacies in the United States, and under prescription in Australia. It was never my belief or the belief of anyone I had been in contact with that it was an anabolic substance. I had always thought it was part of the herbal group of remedies and came from yams.

A week or so later I opened the mail at home. There was a letter from the AFL. That itself wasn't altogether unusual — players often receive letters from the League. But usually they were sent to the club. For it to be sent to my home address was odd. As I read it, I almost fell over. I was being charged under the AFL's Anti-Doping Code.

The letter from Ian Collins, dated 20 April 1998, began:

Please be advised that this acts as an 'Infraction Notice' relative to item 10 of Section 23 of the AFL Anti-

> Doping Code in which the AFL General Manager —
> Football Operations believes on grounds other than
> receiving notification from the Australian Sports Drug
> Agency (ASDA) of a positive test result in which there
> may have been committed a doping offence.

I was told I would be required to attend a hearing of the AFL Tribunal in Melbourne on 29 April at 6pm. It would be held 'in camera' — the press and other people normally permitted to attend such hearings would not be present. I would be allowed legal representation, which was also contrary to normal procedure.

I was dumbfounded. This was something I'd never even contemplated. The worst outcome I'd considered during the many hours I'd spent pondering my situation was not being allowed to take DHEA. I was in a state of panic. To be accused of a doping offence is the worst slur possible for a professional athlete. I knew I'd done nothing wrong. All I'd ever done was pursue a decent quality of life. Football was secondary. If I'd never played again after 1995 it wouldn't have been the end of the world. My 'new' world had begun the previous September when my first child, daughter Madison, was born. For her father to be branded a drug cheat was impossible to comprehend.

The club were good about it. They put my mind at ease as best they could by quickly organising a defence team. They engaged top Melbourne lawyer David Galbally, a long-time friend of Andrew Ireland, to handle the case. He and his colleagues began getting everything together. The board agreed to meet the costs.

All the advice was positive. We were confident that the case wouldn't even get to the tribunal; we thought the AFL would see reason and withdraw the charge. In hindsight, I still believe that had DHEA been part of a more recognised and accepted CFS treatment the charge would have been withdrawn. The air of uncertainty about the whole thing worked against me. As it turned out, our confidence was misplaced. The charge was not withdrawn.

So unknown to everyone outside the inner circle of the club and the AFL, I flew to Melbourne on the morning of Thursday, 7 May 1998 to face the tribunal. Already the hearing had been deferred eight days from the original date following a submission from our legal team. As well as me, the Brisbane contingent included Chairman Noel Gordon, CEO Andrew Ireland and Communications Manager Peter Blucher. We met Galbally and his team at his Queen Street offices to discuss strategy. Everything was going along smoothly — until suddenly the phones started ringing. Not just one. All the mobiles in the room were going off. And not just once. The word was out.

For more than two months the story had been kept quiet; we had been saying nothing, of course, as we were busy preparing the case. But on the day I was to appear, the media got wind of it. And once the secrecy net had been broken there were people we had to talk to.

Andrew rang the club's major sponsors, Coke and CUB. I asked Peter to ring some personal sponsors on my behalf. And I rang some key family members and friends to let them know what was going on. I wanted to tell people close to me before they heard incorrect reports that I'd tested positive for a banned substance, which is exactly what some sections of the media were saying. It didn't matter to the media that it was wrong. Once the story was out it spread like a bushfire.

The one person I desperately wanted to contact just to make sure she knew what was happening was Peta, but she was on a plane to Melbourne from Brisbane.

I don't know how the story got out. There were some conspiracy theories going around at the time but it might have been as simple as the AFL having to confirm the booking for an in-camera hearing at the Administrative Appeals Tribunal, which just happened to be in the

Herald & Weekly Times Tower at Southbank. In the end, no matter how much I would have preferred it to be kept quiet, there was nothing we could do. It just made getting in and out of the hearing more of an issue.

We left Galbally's offices about 5.15pm for the short drive across town. There was a pack of media waiting outside but we ducked into the underground carpark and went up the goods elevator before anyone could find us. If the issue wasn't so serious, this aspect would have been funny.

Sitting on the tribunal were Brian Collis (chairman), Elaine Canty and Shane Maguire. This first session of the hearing lasted two and a half hours, and was confined largely to legal argument. But it was only the beginning.

While all this was going on I was still playing football. On Saturday 9 May we were scheduled to play St Kilda at Waverley. We were bottom of the ladder with a 1–5 win/loss record; St Kilda were fourth, at 5–1. I wondered how the St Kilda players and fans would react to seeing me. I was hopeful that they'd be all right, but not so naive that I didn't realise there may be a few comments.

On the morning of the game I did my usual spot with 'Coodabeen Champions' on 3AW. It was actually good to be able to talk a little about the banning issue, even if I couldn't be specific. I clarified and corrected the misreporting of two days earlier: I said that I hadn't tested positive to anything and that for legal reasons I couldn't go into any more detail. The boys — Ian Cover, Tony Leonard, Greg Champion, Jeff Richardson and Simon Whelan — were great. They were always good fun and were definitely sympathetic to my situation.

So, too, were the St Kilda people. To the football public I'd doubted, my sincere apologies. They were fantastic. I played at fullback on Jason Heatley, a former Fitzroy triallist, so I spent the entire day in the goal square. For two whole quarters I was within earshot of the Saints cheer squad, and not a nasty word was said. It wasn't until a few years later, when the issue was no longer so serious, that the sleeping jokes started. At the end of the game several St Kilda players made a special effort to offer their support as we walked off. Later, a bunch of people from the St Kilda cheer squad even waited upstairs outside the rooms just to wish me good luck. I really appreciated all the support. I knew I'd done the right thing by drawing the matter to the attention of the AFL, but it was nice to hear some positive reinforcement from outside.

When I got on the team bus to head to the airport I was exhausted. It had been a tough day at the office, but a good day. Jarrod Molloy, in his AFL comeback from a knee reconstruction, had kicked six goals in our victory, including a freakish volley effort over his right shoulder from 15m. Coach John Northey had made special mention of the players' support for me at his post-game media conference. 'It's like a member of the family going through a traumatic experience. Everyone is right behind him and wants to show him as much support as possible. He's been through one hell of a time — and quite probably is still going through it — and the best way for us to support him was to give him something to smile about today,' he said. In the paper the following day there was a big photo of me taken just after the final siren. I had my arms in the air. It was an important win for the club, but an even more important one for me. I'd survived what I thought was going to be a traumatic day.

We were scheduled to return to the tribunal on Wednesday, 13 May, for a second sitting. It lasted five hours, but still the case wasn't anything like over. On 20 May there was another five hours of evidence. On 21 May we started session four at 12 noon, in the hope of getting through it all at a reasonable hour. This was history in itself, I think. The first AFL Tribunal case held during normal working hours! This session finished shortly after

5pm. All evidence and preliminary submissions had now been completed, but the chairman had invited both parties to lodge further written submissions. The hearing was to be reconvened one last time for decision at 5pm on Monday, 25 May. Four days to wait.

On one of the trips to Melbourne for the tribunal hearing I was travelling with Lions teammate Nigel Lappin. He was going to Melbourne to be recognised as the 1998 Australian Asthma Sportsman of the Year, following in the footsteps of such luminaries as cricketing legend Allan Border, fellow AFL stars Paul Kelly and Stephen Kernahan, marathon swimmer Susie Moroney, Olympic hockey gold medallist Katrina Powell, Commonwealth swimming ace Matthew Dunn and former Commonwealth diving champion Jenny Donnet. I couldn't help but see the irony of it all. Nige was being given an award in recognition of his successful fight to achieve athletic excellence despite having a chronic medical condition, and I was going to Melbourne to be interrogated for doing what I considered exactly the same thing.

It had been one of the toughest times of my life. The stress was incredible — I'd lost 5kg since the issue had been identified, and there was no other reason for that. I still couldn't believe I could be found guilty. I hadn't tested positive. I hadn't done anything wrong. All I'd done was follow a prescribed course of medication in my search for a near-normal state of health.

Andrew Ireland, Scott Clayton and Dr Alan Mackenzie gave evidence on my behalf. Also, IOC medical commissioner Dr Ken Fitch, who was an expert in drugs in sport and the West Coast Eagles club doctor. Each witness was questioned by Galbally before being cross-examined by the AFL representative. I was last. This was on the final day, after I'd sat nervously through the whole thing.

Initially, regular AFL Tribunal prosecutor and investigations officer Rick Lewis was going to handle the AFL's case, but after the first hearing he was replaced by solicitor Simon Rofe, the man who had written the AFL Anti-Doping Code. I remember thinking, this is great — not only is he prosecuting the case but he's defending his own drug code. Witnesses for the AFL included Ian Collins, Dr Peter Harcourt, ASDA chief executive Natalie Howson and Australian Olympic Committee medical officer Alf Corrigan.

I wasn't in the witness box long. I told my story again, reinforcing that from the outset I followed the directions of my doctors, club and indeed the AFL procedures in clearing medications as they were prescribed. I reminded them too that I was the one who had come forward despite nothing but negative tests and two years of blood tests confirming the same. Still, it was a harrowing experience; I knew that the case was drawing to a close and that not just my football career but my reputation might depend on what I said.

Galbally had done a fantastic job. He'd collected a vast array of material, including a report titled *DHEA White Paper*, prepared by Natrol (a California-based company that manufactures and distributes dietary supplements), in consultation with the US Drug Enforcement Administration. It stated categorically that DHEA does not promote muscle growth and so is not an anabolic steroid. It described it as a synthetically manufactured dietary supplement that is ingested in order to increase the total dietary intake. The report said, as I'd always believed, that DHEA is a wild yam extract.

There was some colourful stuff going on during the case, too. Two days in, Brisbane's Chairman, Noel Gordon, broke the media comment gag to express the club's disappointment that the matter had become public. A week or so later, Gordon, always passionate about his club and never one to back away from a fight, was in strife again for suggesting in a television interview that the AFL had put undue pressure on Dr Fitch not to appear. The League wasn't happy with him.

My good mate Paul Roos, too, was in trouble. Speaking at an official AFL media conference, he was asked about my case and explained that I had been told by ASDA that I could continue taking DHEA. That was true. It had happened twice when Dr Alan Mackenzie rang the ASDA Hotline on my behalf. Yet Roosy was sent a 'please explain' letter from the AFL: he had to persuade them that he should not be fined $5000 for commenting on a closed tribunal hearing. Happily, sanity prevailed and his fine was waived. Just as well for me, because he would have wanted me to pay it.

On 25 May we headed back to Melbourne. As we waited outside the tribunal room for the final verdict I was as nervous as I've ever been. Probably not quite as nervous as the last person I spoke to on the phone before entering the room. Peta was worse than me.

For some reason, I recall that we started two minutes early. There was no risk of anyone being late. Collis read from a prepared statement. All I wanted to hear were the words 'not guilty'. They didn't come. He went on with a lot of legal jargon and finished with 'not sustained'. I thought I knew what that meant but I wasn't absolutely certain. I looked to my left. Noel Gordon's beaming smile told me I was right. We'd won. I immediately left the room to call Pete. I couldn't let her live a minute longer without knowing the good news.

Relief doesn't come close to describing how I felt. To label a sportsman a possible drug cheat is about the worst thing you can say to them. Now it was as if I'd been vindicated, and everything I'd said privately and publicly throughout the case had been proven correct. It was as if the tribunal was saying, 'This problem is real.' It was a win for CFS sufferers Australia-wide.

We adjourned to the team hotel, the Centra, part of the old World Congress Building, for a hurriedly convened media conference. I told the media that I had always been confident that justice would be done and I'd be cleared, but I also admitted that I may still have to quit football if my health suffered. I told them I hoped to get permission from the AFL to take the medication DHEA, but knew it was not likely I'd get it.

I wanted to stress that DHEA was not a cure for CFS but that I had concluded that DHEA, along with other medications, had had a positive effect on my condition over time. And that was the most important thing. That was what the whole case had been about. Dr Whiting had told me I shouldn't go too long without DHEA, but how long was too long? Days, weeks, months? Nobody could say for sure.

I only knew one thing for sure — my health had deteriorated since I'd stopped taking DHEA, but I couldn't say categorically that that was related to CFS or DHEA. After all, it had been an extraordinarily stressful month and I hadn't had much sleep.

After the media conference I went to the nearby Channel Seven studios at South Melbourne to pre-record that night's edition of *Talking Footy*. Ironically, on the panel alongside host Bruce McAvaney was Leigh Matthews. If he had known then what he knew about four months later, he would have been almost as happy as me. Almost. At least I hope so! He was going to be my coach in 1999.

Then I caught up with the Brisbane contingent for an overdue dinner at the Emerald Hotel in Clarendon Street. It was a favourite watering hole of Gordon and Ireland, and even though it was late they knew we could get a good steak. I even allowed myself one light beer before heading off.

I stayed that night with Peta at the home of Fitzroy ex-teammate Paul Broderick, who was now playing at

Richmond. Pete and Madison had been there throughout the trial. They'd travelled to Melbourne for the start, not expecting for one second that it would last 19 days, but Pete wasn't going to go home until it was over. She did it pretty tough, because she knew what a guilty verdict would have done to me. As often happens, it's the person closest to the person under the spotlight who carries the most stress. The Brodericks were just sensational. Nothing was ever a problem, and never was I going to be anything but cleared. Each time I visited Melbourne for another session of the hearing I stayed there, too; the Fitzroy connection lives on.

Most of the media had been pretty good throughout the case in what they said and wrote. We'd had a weekly battle getting into the tribunal building — after the first session, they got a lot smarter. They would stake out each of the entry points, so we'd have to push our way through hordes of television cameras going in and coming out. I guess they were only doing their job, but it definitely got a bit tedious.

I tried not to read too much of the press during the tribunal hearing. All I was interested in was the verdict. It was a 12-page document signed by Brian Collis, Elaine Canty and Shane Maguire, and it said, in summary:

Alastair Lynch did not act in breach of the AFL Anti-Doping Code as at all times he acted bona fide in accordance with and in reliance upon what he reasonably and understandably believed to be the advice of an independent organization he was directed to make enquiries to as to whether he could or could not take a particular substance.

The tribunal members went to great lengths to emphasise that my case should not be seen as a precedent. It was unique, dependent upon a number of particular facts and circumstances. Fair enough.

Essentially, the whole matter revolved around the uncertainties about CFS. What is it? What causes it? How do you treat it?

If the medical fraternity and the greater population in general had known what CFS was and how to cure it in 1998, my doping case would never have happened. I wouldn't have been in a position where my integrity was questioned.

I stopped taking DHEA the day the AFL denied my application. And I've never taken it since. Happily, concern that my health would suffer badly without DHEA turned out to be unfounded. There was no guarantee that this would happen, just as there was no guarantee about anything else to do with treatment of CFS. Dr Whiting had merely been trying to cover all the bases.

If my health had nosedived badly without DHEA I would have retired. Now, even in retirement, I'm happy not to use it — as long as I don't need it. If things were to get so bad that it was necessary to take it again, I'd have no hesitation doing so. As I stressed throughout the case, it was all about quality of life, about being able to do what normal people do. I hope it never again gets to that stage.

Countless people said to me at the time that I could have kept taking DHEA, and it's a line that has often been repeated since. And they're right. Nobody would have known. But it's not the way I live. I'd only be cheating myself. If I was a cheat, I wouldn't have told anyone at the outset that I was taking what I'd just found out was a banned substance. I told the AFL because it was the right thing to do. I did so because I believed I needed to take DHEA to enjoy a reasonable quality of life. Football wasn't the only consideration. If I could play without it and still enjoy good health it would be a bonus. But, in keeping with the advice I had received from Dr

Whiting, I believed I would be better off taking DHEA. That's why I made an application to keep using it.

In researching this book I tracked down Dr Whiting. He'd gone into semi-retirement for about two years from December 2001 due to sheer exhaustion, but is now back doing some part-time consultancy — and is again too busy to take on new patients.

I wasn't surprised to learn from him that DHEA is now the number one agent for treating the 'millions and millions' of CFS sufferers worldwide. As he suspected, it has now been proven that it helps the immune system, sleep, cognition, blood pressure and bowel function. It also helps reduce — and in some cases eliminate — muscle pain and headaches, and chronic infection.

Over the years, as my condition improved, I saw less and less of the specialists and their new treatments, so it was pleasing, I guess, to hear Dr Whiting say that the publicity my condition attracted helped increase the legitimacy of CFS in Australia and so helped a lot of people. It was even more pleasing to learn that CFS treatment had progressed enormously and that now CFS isn't quite the same long-term sentence it used to be.

It was interesting to catch up with Dr Whiting. He had been so good to me. Seven days before his second wedding, for example, he had dropped everything to fit in an after-hours consultation. He even gave me a blood test form and suggested I might like to see exactly how my levels had changed. I might do it, too, just out of curiosity.

9

RELAPSE AND REBIRTH

If there's one thing I learned about CFS, it is that you should never underestimate it. Never think you've got it beaten. Not totally. Even when you're feeling terrific you need to be mindful that it can bite back at any moment. Just when you least expect it. Just as it did to me in February 1999.

For the first time since 1994 I was feeling on top of the world. I'd done pretty much a full pre-season campaign and was fitter and stronger than I'd been for five years. And I was really excited. Leigh Matthews, the greatest player of all time, had been appointed Brisbane Lions coach. We couldn't have asked for a better man. As a playing group we were screaming out for something positive to hang on to after the troubles of 1998. Just by walking in the door he lifted the spirits of the place immeasurably.

Unbeknown to any of us at the time, Matthews had agreed to take the Brisbane coaching job on the afternoon of our Round 22 game against St Kilda in 1998. He was in Brisbane on television duty, and sat in the commentary box that night knowing he was watching the side he would take over. He wouldn't have been particularly impressed with what he saw, but everyone knew we were better than we'd shown in 1998.

Matthews' appointment represented a chance for everyone at the Lions to make a fresh start after the nightmare that was 1998. A chance to put behind us a year in which my co-captain Michael Voss had broken his leg, John Northey had been sacked mid-year, caretaker coach Roger Merrett had not been reappointed and we had suffered untold off-field turmoil.

The first time Leigh addressed the players was on the day his appointment was announced — Tuesday, 7 September 1998. I remember thinking how calm and considered he was. I'd heard stories of how he used to lose the plot when he coached Collingwood and fly off the handle, but in six years playing under him I never really witnessed anything like that.

From day one Leigh had the entire playing group eating out of his hand. Even before we met him as a coach he had an aura about him which demanded total respect. He immediately got everyone heading in the same direction. He had such a presence — and, not that he needed it, a remarkable capacity to sell his message. He didn't come in with a big fist. He just promised a fresh start for everyone. What had happened previously didn't matter, he said. Everyone would start with a clean slate. And, not for the first time, we heard one of his favourite sayings — players play, coaches coach, management manages and directors direct. That's the way it was going to be.

There was one promise: that the Lions would have the best off-field support network in the competition. There would be no excuses. Anything and everything we needed to perform as a football department would be there. And at the top of the list was a medical staff second to none. There was no point having the best team in the country if every third player spent half the year on the injured list, he said.

There was another rule he established from day one — if a team meeting is scheduled to start at 5pm, don't bother arriving at 5.01pm, he told us. The door would be shut and you'd sit outside until afterwards. A little thing, but a sign that he meant business. There were no shortcuts and near enough was never going to be good enough. He established a code of behaviour built around commonsense, courtesy and punctuality. It was all about treating people the right way in the hope and expectation that others would do likewise. A pretty good starting point.

I'd met Leigh socially a couple of times before his appointment but I'd never really got to know him. A lot of the younger blokes found him intimidating, which was understandable. After all, he had been voted the best player of the 20th century. But I found him easy to talk to — perhaps because I was a bit older and was co-captain of the club. He was easy-going, enthusiastic and encouraging. Before he went to Ireland to coach the Australian International Rules team he even asked my opinion on my old Fitzroy teammate and housemate Matty Armstrong when he was putting together his coaching structure. Somehow 'Dogsy' got the job anyway.

There was a bright and fresh feeling around the club. After consolidating years in 1997 and 1998 in which I was happy just to get back on the paddock and make a half-reasonable contribution, I really felt ready to go in 1999. I felt I could really make a genuine impact. Even get back to my very best. I was training twice a day with the team and doing the majority of the running; certainly all the running the big fellas were doing. I was really fit. I used to drive home at night looking forward to the next day when I could get back for more. At last, I felt that CFS was behind me.

In mid-February we hit an extremely hot period. But I was feeling fine. I kept pushing. One day at Coorparoo we had a very hard running session. Michael McLean, a former teammate who had returned to the club as an assistant coach, even said to me, 'Are you sure you should be doing this? Don't you want to take it easy?'

Driving home I didn't feel quite right. Something was wrong. Almost overnight my sleep patterns went haywire. The muscle fatigue which had plagued me for so many years returned. I had the aches and pains, especially in my legs. I'd taken a massive step backwards, and all the hard work and progress I'd made in the last four months on the track was lost.

Lesson learned the hard way: never, ever, underestimate CFS.

I missed a practice match against Sydney at Campbelltown. This wasn't something I'd ordinarily remember, but Matthews, who lived on the opposite side of town, dropped in to my place on his way home from the airport to see how I was. Apparently we'd really struggled up forward that day, so he was keen to see when I might be right. It was a terrific gesture. I knew then and there that we had the right coach. Sadly, I wasn't going to be able to help him for a while.

I missed the first two months of the season. First with CFS and later with a hamstring problem. I'd overdone the work, and in the stinging heat it had flattened me. It was going to be a slow process back. Patience, again, had become my greatest ally, and this time I wasn't about to rush things.

I was feeling pretty sorry for myself, but it wasn't long before I got a reminder that it wasn't the end of the world.

In Round 1, Leigh Matthews' first game as Brisbane Lions coach, we played St Kilda at the Gabba. I was sitting in the dugout between the two coaches' benches, down in front of the old Lions Social Club. Next to me was ruck coach and ex-teammate Damian Bourke. It was a night game but it was still stinking hot. I remember saying, 'Look at Muz — he's doing it tough.'

Muz was our head trainer, Murray Johnson. A terrific old fella who typified the backroom boys who gave so much of their time for little or no reward, just to be a part of the club. The players just love the trainers, strappers, rubbers, water carriers, even the statisticians and general helpers. Sometimes we take them for granted, but that doesn't mean we don't actually appreciate what they do. They are one of the few constants about football clubs — they are all fantastic.

About halfway through the final quarter Muz collapsed right out in front of where Bourkey and I were sitting. It's something I'll never forget. As it turned out, it wasn't a heart attack but a heart arrest, when oxygen wasn't getting to his brain. It could have killed him. First to him was Lions runner Robert Dickson, who in 2002 would win national notoriety — and $500,000 — via Channel Nine's *Survivor* program. Fortunately, Dicko was a trained National Safety Council helicopter pilot. He was an expert in first-aid procedures and performed mouth to mouth. Next to reach Muz was Ian Stone, the St Kilda doctor. I only knew him because he was an ex-Fitzroy doctor. Then came the Brisbane doctors and the St John's ambulance officer.

Twice the big heart of old Muz stopped beating as they fought for 30 minutes on the boundary line to save his life. Luckily, he wouldn't give in. And between him and the expert team of medics, with some help from oxygen, heart massage and a zap from the defibrillator, they got his ticker going again and he pulled through. He was even conscious enough as they took him away in an ambulance to apologise for all the fuss. Typical Muz. He underwent a triple heart bypass on 1 April and was back on duty before we knew it, though he was confined to the bench for a while.

We beat St Kilda by 89 points, but it didn't seem so important that night. I didn't feel quite so sorry for myself as I went home. My health wasn't great, but at least I was alive. And for 10 minutes I had feared that a true gentleman wasn't going to be able to say the same thing.

Under Leigh Matthews the club had employed an entirely new medical team. They were fantastic, and would become key elements in the success that was to follow. Physiotherapists Peter Stanton and Victor Popov and doctors Andrew Smith and Paul McConnell would work closely with ex-Collingwood and Brisbane player Craig Starcevich, one of the few key off-field football people from the Northey/Merrett era who had survived. Still on deck, too, was surgeon Jim Fardoulys, although happily I managed not to need his services. Soon they were joined by strength coach Scott Murphy. A premiership medical team if ever there has been one.

They set up their operation in the medical clinic at the Gabba, upstairs from the players' facilities. It was the best thing I'd seen. A real one-stop shop. Anything and everything we needed in a medical sense was there. Even a 25m two-lane lap pool. AFL football had gone to the next level with professionalism.

It was through the Lions' medical family that I met Howard Arbuthnot. He organised the club's compulsory massage program: each player was required to have two deep tissue massages a week. It was part of the overall maintenance program to try to prevent injuries before they happened. We had 10 massage therapists who would come into the club twice a week with their portable massage tables and spend about 45 minutes per player. Each one worked with the same group of players each week. This was important, because they got to know the players' bodies — where the problem spots were and what each one needed to keep him in good working order.

Howard was a former Queensland pole-vaulting champion who had worked with the Australian medical team at the 1992, 1996 and 2000 Olympic Games. He was my personal masseur and I was his No. 1 patient. I saw him at least twice a week in season from the start of 1999 until the end of my career. He had a fair old battle keeping me on the track.

With the return of my CFS I also went to a specialist at the Wesley Hospital. He did repeated muscle biopsies from samples taken from my thigh and skin biopsies from my forearm as part of an ongoing campaign to find a biological reason for my condition. It was an endless program. I just kept hoping that there would be a medical breakthrough and suddenly we'd find the answer.

I played two games in the reserves before returning to AFL football: one low-key effort against Labrador at the Gabba, then four full-tempo 10-minute bursts against Broadbeach at the Gold Coast. I kicked eight goals, which was a good confidence booster. I returned to the seniors in Round 9, and though I didn't miss another game, I still wasn't right. I struggled all year. In fact I was a long way short of the mark. I was still paying for my over-exuberance during the pre-season.

Though my energy levels were low and my post-game recovery was slow, my biggest problem was sleeping. This was phase two of CFS: I'd gone through the stage of not being able to stay awake, and now I was in the opposite cycle. I'd tried various sleeping tablets over the years and one by one I'd become immune to them. I'd go two and three nights without any real sleep. It was killing me. Even if I'd get to sleep it would be shallow sleep. I'd wake up all the time and struggle to get back to sleep. Sometimes I slept so lightly that I'd wake up unsure if I'd really been asleep. I'd even tried hypnosis, but without any luck.

After back-to-back visits to Adelaide in Rounds 18 and 19 I was feeling shocking. I'd started on the interchange bench against the Crows in the second game of the Football Park double-header and was to play as a ruckman. Midway through the first quarter I relieved Matty Clarke, but by the time I ran to the centre of the ground I was gone. I spent most of the rest of the night on the bench.

We were desperate for answers. Football Manager Graeme 'Gubby' Allan had arranged for me to fly from Adelaide to Sydney to see two specialists. I can't remember their names and there weren't any great answers. What was important to me was the support from the club that this represented. Leigh, Gubby and the new-look medical team didn't know the full background to my illness and obviously hadn't experienced the previous four years with me. They could easily have thrown their hands up in the air. But they didn't. They were incredibly sympathetic and supportive. They set out to learn as much as they could about the best way to manage my CFS. Without their efforts I would have been finished. Instead, I was able to play five more years and savour three wonderful premierships. So please excuse me if I get a little over-indulgent when it comes to talking about these people.

It's interesting nowadays to talk to Gubby about that 48 hours in Sydney. He admits that it 'shocked him', and proved 'a real eye-opener'. And though he says it was part of the job, and he did it out of a sense of duty and responsibility, it was more important to me than that. It convinced me that I had an ally in the football manager, and I felt that through his experience, others in the football operation became more knowledgeable. I never felt Leigh and Gubby doubted me, but to have a positive show of support at that difficult time was tremendous.

One of the main things that kept me going through the tough times was the commitment of the medical team to find a better way to deal with my condition. Together, we tried something new all the time. We realised that I didn't have to be the fittest player in the competition — just fit enough to play a role at full forward, to provide a marking target and a contest in the scoring zone. If I was feeling well, my general fitness would be enough to get me through, and would allow me to play at the extremities of the ground. I'd play mostly at full forward, with an occasional run at fullback when we needed a specific match-up.

Also, we learned how to manage things much better and conserve energy. We identified what worked and what didn't work. It was a process of elimination. We had already learned one big lesson: early season heat was out. The other lesson we learned, though more slowly, was that long travel was also out. We didn't see it that year — I'd missed the two early season trips to Perth because of my CFS relapse.

At least I was playing. In Round 21 we beat Melbourne by 55 points at the MCG. I kicked the first and last goals but didn't do a lot in between in what was my 200th game. Tim Notting kicked a career-best six goals and I managed to be nowhere near a melee which cost Michael Voss, Nigel Lappin, Darryl White, Simon Black and Matthew Kennedy a combined $8500. It was Brisbane's second win in 16 visits to the MCG during my time with the club — it was nice to change things around.

Round 22 was another milestone game. Not for me, but for the Collingwood Football Club. It was their last game at Victoria Park, the Magpies' home of 107 years. The security was increased in expectation of trouble but there was no sign of anything untoward. It was more a party, especially after we got right on top early.

I used to like playing at Victoria Park. At times it was a bit of an adventure, but it was a tremendous place to play. It was full of history and tradition. The spectators were always close to the players, which ensured a good atmosphere, and you rarely failed to get a full house when you visited the Magpies. They were the tribal enemy of Fitzroy, but even if the crowd is barracking against you, it's better to have noise and atmosphere than empty stands and silence. It was a typical suburban ground. Sadly, by 1999 they were a fast disappearing commodity in AFL football. I'd also played in the last game at St Kilda's old home ground at Moorabbin in 1992, when the Saints beat Fitzroy 14.18 (102) to 10.24 (84) in Round 20.

My favourite ground in Melbourne was always Princes Park. I played a lot of football there and I liked the dimensions of the place, and the fact that, as with all the suburban grounds, the crowd was close. It's a shame to see these grounds being phased out of AFL football, but I guess that's the price you pay for progress. It's all about providing quality facilities for all concerned, and the most economical way to do that is to have fewer grounds which more teams play at.

For obvious reasons the Gabba became a favourite, too. The support I always got there was nothing short of sensational — except, perhaps, when I visited Brisbane twice as a member of the enemy with Fitzroy.

My first visit to the Gabba was on a Sunday afternoon in July 1991. It was then a peculiar shape, with a big pocket at one end and no pocket at the other end. And it had a greyhound track around the outside, between the playing arena and the people. We got changed in the cricket dressing rooms, which were so small you almost had to go outside to change your mind. The Bears gave Fitzroy a 65 point flogging, with Cameron O'Brien kicking six goals and Brad Hardie five.

It's hard to believe that from humble beginnings as an AFL ground came one of the great football venues. By the time I returned, in Round 6, 1993 — this time for a 27 point loss — the redevelopment had begun. The dog track had gone and even for the visitors the player facilities were good. And the hotch-potch of grandstands had begun their transformation into the magnificent arena of today.

Every ground had its own feel, and I liked those with some real history to them. Like the MCG and the SCG — growing up in Tasmania I saw a lot of the Swans at the SCG on television on a Sunday afternoon. I also liked the

WACA. The surface was always like a bowling green, and for some reason Fitzroy, even when we were struggling, always tended to play well over there.

Different grounds presented different challenges. When you went to Geelong's Kardinia Park or Footscray's Whitten Oval you had to adopt a different game plan as a key forward because the ground was so much longer than most. This was in total contrast to short grounds like the SCG. There weren't any grounds I didn't like; if you're going to play AFL football you play whenever and wherever, and you don't worry about anything except the contest.

In September 1999 we came dreadfully close to winning the AFL flag. We'd finished third at the end of the home-and-away season, belted Carlton by 73 points and then beat the Western Bulldogs by 53 points at the Gabba in the semi-finals. All of a sudden we'd won 10 in a row and were within a game of the grand final. It was North Melbourne at the MCG in the preliminary final. Again.

It wasn't to be our year. Chris Scott and Craig McRae missed through suspension for what were pretty minor incidents against the Dogs, Michael Voss was already out with an ankle problem and we lost Simon Black after five minutes to a fractured eye socket. We led at half-time in what had been a really courageous effort, but we were just undermanned and ended up losing by 45 points. A week later the Kangaroos posted a 35-point grand final win over Carlton, whom we'd beaten so comprehensively at the start of the finals. Yet we'd gone from wooden-spooners to fourth in 12 months. An amazing turnaround on and off the field for our club.

If there was any period of complacency in the Lions ranks during my six years under Leigh Matthews it came in season 2000. Coming off a fantastic 1999 we struggled to find any sort of consistency. We didn't lose more than two in a row for the whole year, but we didn't win more than two in a row either, until the last four games of the home-and-away season. We eventually got ourselves into a position to mount a challenge, finishing sixth at the end of the home-and-away campaign with a 12–10 record, but it was a year in which it didn't really happen for us.

The season proper hadn't even started when Leigh Matthews stamped his authority on 2000: he told me I couldn't play in Round 1, against Carlton at Optus Oval. The Friday was an absolute stinker, temperature-wise, and that evening he discussed the idea of leaving me out with the assistant coaches. I got the message that if it stayed really hot I wouldn't be playing. On Saturday morning I bumped into him in the lift in the team hotel. 'You're not playing,' he told me. It was a good call. I knew I had to be careful, but it's one thing to know it and another thing to do it. I would have been silly enough to play, because I didn't want to let my coach and my teammates down. I would have hoped it might have been one of those days where you get through all right, the ball bounces your way a couple of times and no damage is done.

Halfway through the last quarter I was pleased that the coach had overruled me. I saw Michael Voss, who is a super runner, heading towards the Heatley Stand end and he was almost delirious. When I talked to the players afterwards, they suggested that I would have died. And while perhaps they were being a little melodramatic, I got the message. Even people who had been sitting on the interchange bench looking into the sun were nursing major sunburn. I was pleased the coach had been strong enough to make the call. Carlton flogged us anyway, and my presence wouldn't have altered the result, so it just meant that I didn't tempt fate in the heat as I'd done a little over 12 months earlier.

More importantly, we were sticking to our medical plan. We'd formulated an approach to managing my CFS which we were comfortable with, though we didn't know for certain whether or not it was going to work. Yet we had to stick to it. Thanks to the strong mind of the coach and the medical staff, we did.

I was back the following week and very pleased about it. Why? Because it was a historic moment in AFL football. The Lions played the Western Bulldogs in the first 'indoor' AFL premiership game — under the roof of what was then known as Colonial Stadium, now Telstra Dome. And I got to toss the coin on this momentous occasion.

Michael Voss and I were, of course, co-captains, and we used a very deep and involved process to determine who would toss the coin — scissors, paper, rock. I won, so I got the job. I even called correctly against Bulldogs skipper Scott Wynd. It was legitimate, which is more than I can say for a funny occasion when I shared the coin toss with Carlton's Stephen Kernahan at Optus Oval in Round 11, 1997.

Tina Arena had tossed the coin, and as the visiting captain, I called. 'Heads,' I said. I looked down to see a tail. Seeing no reaction from the Blues skipper, I quickly pointed one way and ran off. After the final team huddle I finished up directly opposed to Kernahan, who plays wearing contact lenses. Just before the first bounce I said

to him, 'You do realise it was a tail, don't you?' To which
he replied, 'Damn, that's the second time I've done that.
Don't tell anyone.' Sorry, 'Sticks'!

Playing indoors was different. We were used to a blue
sky as the backdrop for the ball in the air, and inside
Colonial we had a roof as the backdrop instead. It
changed our depth perception. I'm not sure if it was better
or worse — it probably depended on whether I was having
a good day or a bad day — but it was noticeably different.

I loved playing inside. Without the interference of the
elements the game was really fast and the ball zipped from
end to end more quickly than usual. And you didn't need a
massive crowd to have a really good atmosphere. I remember
hoping when the plans for the stadium were released a
couple of years earlier that I'd be playing long enough to
sample it. Happily, I still had a little extra time up my sleeve.

I played a pretty fair 2000 and kicked 68 goals. At the
time, this was an equal career best. More important to me,
though, was the fact that Daniel Bradshaw (56) and Luke
Power (52) also topped the half-century. It was only the
eighth time in history that three players on the same team
had kicked 50-plus goals in the same season, and it
underlined the potential of those two outstanding young
players. Braddy was in his fifth season already at 21, and

'Finger' was in his third season at 20. Finger? It's Luke's nickname because he's missing part of a finger on his left hand.

Sadly, both of them were missing when our season came to a halt against Carlton at the MCG on semi-final day. Luke and I had bagged five goals apiece in a 34-point qualifying final win over the Bulldogs at the Gabba, but he missed out against the Blues because of a hamstring injury. Braddy was an altogether different story, a story which catapulted the media-shy boy from Wodonga into the national spotlight.

Daniel and girlfriend Angie were expecting their first child. She'd been away for a couple of weeks, spending time with her mother, and when the Lions flew to Melbourne she dropped into the team hotel on the Friday night to catch up with him. About 10pm she left, and soon after her waters broke. The father-to-be told the hierarchy what had happened and raced up to the hospital. He sat there for an hour or so before he was sent back to the hotel. Being a first child, the odds were that it would be a long labour. Best get some sleep, they told him. They'd ring if anything happened.

Back at the hotel he somehow managed to do as they suggested, but before 7am he was on the phone to the hospital. Still no baby, but he knew he had a decision to make. He contacted Shane Johnson, officially the club's player development manager but known to the players as the first person you call when you've got a problem. Then Leigh Matthews came to his room. The coach's advice was simple — you've got to do what you've got to do. Braddy was off: the birth of his first child took priority over a football match. Emergency player Marcus Picken was enjoying breakfast when he got the tap on the shoulder. He was in.

Jake Bradshaw was born at 3.40pm on 19 September 2000, about halfway through the third quarter of the semi-final. By that time we were long gone. Carlton beat us by 82 points. Another year down. It was my 13th in the AFL if you include 1995, and I'd played 226 games. I was still conscious of my CFS and careful not to overdo things, yet I felt as well as I had for a long time.

I was worried, though. I was starting to wonder if my football dream had passed me by. Twice the Bears/Lions had reached the preliminary final — in 1996 and 1999 — and now we'd slipped again. A lot of teams don't get another chance. In recent years Melbourne, Geelong, Sydney, Western Bulldogs, Richmond and St Kilda had fallen when they'd been agonisingly close, getting within a game of the grand final but not able to take that last step. Certainly, we were at the crossroads: could we capitalise on what we knew was a talented playing list, capable of going all the way, or would we continue to struggle? If I knew then what I knew later, and that Leigh Matthews would find a perfect route through the times ahead, I would have enjoyed the off-season a lot more.

10

THE TURNING POINT

Deep in the bowels of the Richard Pratt Stand at Optus
Oval, Carlton, is a small room which measures 3m x 4m.
It's made of big cement blocks, has a whiteboard on the
front wall, three levels of tiered timber bench seating in
the back, and grey carpet on the floor, and it goes by the
name of the coach's meeting room in the visitors' dressing
rooms. It's hardly the most impressive facility I've been in,
but it was a special place in my career. And not just
because it was there that I had to sheepishly knock on the
door when I was late for the coach's pre-game address on
the day of my first reserves game at Fitzroy in 1988.

It was on Saturday, 19 May 2001, in this nondescript

little room that the transformation of the Brisbane Lions from a good side to a great side began. This was a metamorphosis that would establish our side as what many experts have described as the greatest side of all time. And certainly give me the highlight of my career — three premierships.

On this typical overcast Melbourne afternoon I walked into the rooms devastated. We'd been hammered by Carlton by 74 points; utterly humiliated and embarrassed. For a side which was supposedly among the better ones in the competition, having finished fourth and fifth in the two previous years, it was a pathetic effort. About as bad as I can recall for my entire career.

But coach Leigh Matthews didn't scream or explode. Instead, he set in train some serious self-assessment of exactly where we were at and how we were going about our football. And he told us, bluntly, that if we continued to play in that manner we were on a highway to nowhere. He was right.

It had been a bad day all round. Small forwards Luke Power and Craig McRae had been ruled unfit, joining Shaun Hart on the casualty list, so we were savagely depleted at ground level in the forward line. We opted to go in with three ruckmen, Clark Keating, Beau McDonald and Trent Knobel, plus Matthew Kennedy and Darryl White, who could be used as ruckmen at a pinch.

We were taught a lesson in team football by a Carlton side coached by my first AFL coach, David Parkin. They played for each other. They played as a team. And they did all the little team things that, when there isn't a lot between the two sides, make the difference. They were fantastic.

For pure talent, outsiders might say the Lions were a better side. Yet as a team on the day the Blues were much better. The lesson was simple. The Carlton players, with a 4–3 win/loss record going into the game, and equal with us on the ladder, were prepared to sacrifice individual statistics and personal recognition for the team good. To make sure that the ball was in the hands of their better players like Anthony Koutoufides, Scott Camporeale, Craig Bradley and Brett Ratten. It didn't matter who kicked the goals, as long as someone did.

We were about as low as we could go. It wasn't the biggest loss I played in but it was as bad as any because of the way we went about it. We were supposed to win, but we were never really in the contest, and were totally exposed by the Blues: 9.14 (68) to 21.16 (142).

However, this experience underlined just how quickly things can turn around if you get everything in order. Two weeks later we started a 16-game winning streak that would take us all the way to football's greatest triumph — a premiership.

The 30 minutes we spent behind those closed doors, just the coach and 22 players, were the making of a playing group that would go on to win three consecutive flags.

On the Monday, Leigh Matthews rang some of the team leaders. I was at Indooroopilly Shoppingtown when he rang me, and we talked for the best part of half an hour. On the Tuesday, in our weekly review meeting, he put in place a system that would transform our approach.

Each player was allocated a specific role within the team structure. Almost like a job description. And it was his responsibility to fulfil that role: nothing more, nothing less. No worrying about other players and what they were doing. All each player had to do was do his own job.

Not everyone was going to get the glamour roles that would see them finishing at the top of the statistics sheet or receiving huge media plaudits. And this was the most important thing: that didn't matter. What mattered was the fact that the team would benefit.

The players who set up a goal were just as important as the player who kicked the goal. And so were the players who delivered the ball to the player who kicked the ball.

And just as important, if not more important, were the players who were prepared to make a sacrifice — and whose work would generally go unnoticed. The player who would deliberately lead away from the ball just to drag his opponent away and create extra space for the target players to work in, for instance. The fact that he was never going to get the ball didn't matter. Or the player who maintained maximum defensive pressure by chasing and chasing his opponent. Again, it didn't matter whether or not he caught his man. The willingness to keep chasing every time was what mattered, because the one time he caught him and forced a turnover might help create the one goal that made the difference.

It was about sacrifice and discipline. Or, as the coach would say, about investing in the team. Being prepared to accept an outwardly lesser role for the good of the group.

It was about predictability. If everyone knew what everyone else was going to do we would become a very predictable side. And a very efficient side. It would breed confidence and elevate performance.

As the coach said, time and again, we had to understand the plan, embrace the plan and execute the plan. And not just 19 or 20 of us. It was always going to take 22 players to be totally committed to the plan every time we played, realising that with team success the individual would be rewarded.

For me, predictable meant always being 15m from goal, at the top of the goal square. Not always to take the mark and not even always to be the target. But always to provide a contest whenever the opportunity presented itself. So we could build our forward line entries around getting the ball in long and quick to the hot spot, and so that the smaller players like Craig McRae knew where the ball was going. And where they had to get to.

I had a close on-field relationship with McRae, or 'Fly'. It was essential between a marking forward and crumbing forward. He'd know exactly where I was going to be when the ball came in long and direct, and what I'd do if I couldn't mark the ball. And he'd know where I was going to be whenever he got the ball. In time this all became so predictable that we didn't even need to communicate by voice. It was instinctive; it just happened.

For someone like Daniel Bradshaw, who would often line up beside me deep inside the forward 50m zone, predictable meant always leading out from the square, and always making sure he dragged his opponent with him. If he was clear and in a good position, the ball-carrier would deliver him the ball. If not, they could go long and direct to the top of the square. That was the team plan.

For midfielders, it meant not having to think when they were sending the ball forward under pressure. At times, sure, they could pick out a free teammate or Braddy. But if there was nothing else on, or they were under pressure, they knew they could always go long and direct to the top of the square, because there would be a contest.

Also, for midfielders, it meant being disciplined enough not to run forward and try to take a contested mark inside the forward 50m. They had to trust the designated forward–50 players to do that. And they had to help create space inside the forward–50 by making sure their opponents weren't there.

You had to trust your teammates. You had to have faith in the plan. And that was one of Leigh Matthews' great strengths. No matter what it was, and what its origins, he had a great ability to sell the idea. Each player walked away from that initial meeting totally convinced it was the way to go.

There was always a lot of positive reinforcement. We talked about it often. At the Friday night planning meeting before every game we'd commit to the team plan. We'd talk about individual roles so as to reinforce it. At the Tuesday review meeting after every game we'd make special mention of selfless contributions of all the players who had played their role.

The player who put a shepherd on for a player kicking a goal was just as important as the player who kicked the goal, and as the one who passed the goal-kicker the ball. And as the one who, five play-phases back, won possession in a one-on-one contest at the other end of the ground.

All this helped create an enormous team-first ethos. And with it came a deep-seated desire not just to respect the contribution of your teammates but to make sure you didn't let your teammates down by going outside your role and against the team plan.

It sounds corny, but it was exactly like the chain being only as strong as its weakest link. That really was the principle on which the Lions' assault on the 2001 AFL premiership and subsequent premierships was built that day at Carlton.

The 'play your role' mindset didn't have quite as immediate an impact as it might have. The following week we lost by five points to Adelaide at the Gabba. Marcus Picken, in what would be his last game for the club, had a 75m shot after the siren to win. An impossible task, and it fell short. But it was a much improved team performance. A lot of good signs. Most importantly, there was a willingness among the playing group to try to do what was being asked.

The following week was a huge week in the evolution of the Brisbane Lions. Essendon, premiers of 2000 and clearly the best side in the League at the time, were coming to the Gabba.

Collectively, they looked unbeatable. But the new team-first, role-playing mindset made it easier for us to believe that we could beat them. We didn't worry about beating this supposedly impregnable Essendon machine as a whole. We worried about our one-on-one match-up. Could we beat our opponent? Or, if we weren't having the best of days, could we continue to do as the team plan commanded? Could we do the little things — provide a contest where it was expected? Maintain maximum defensive pressure?

If you'd asked any player, 'Can we beat Essendon?' he'd have been realistic and said, 'Well, they are a super side, but we'll have a crack and I think we're a good chance.' But if you had asked them, 'Can you beat your opponent?' it would have been simple. 'Yes,' they'd have said. We broke it down into 22 individual match-ups. And suddenly our confidence levels were much higher.

We didn't worry about the result; we focused on the process. Each player would just go out to do his job. He'd trust the bloke next to him to do his job, too. And the bloke next to him. And if everyone did that, the bottom line would look after itself.

Leigh Matthews helped, with a line which has become part of football folklore: 'If it bleeds you can kill it,' he told the media. It was a line borrowed from the Arnold Schwarzenegger movie *Predator*, and it was exactly what we were all about — beating the unbeatable. Leigh had actually dropped it on the players in the review meeting a few days earlier and got a good response, so I wasn't surprised to see him trot it out publicly. He loved that sort of thing, and was always conscious of the need to help promote the game, especially in the Queensland market, so he was quick to seize on a good one-liner.

Looking back on it, it's really quite incredible. We didn't lose another game for the year. We won 16 in a row to go all the way. Appropriately, it was a streak that began and ended with Essendon, who had gone into the season with people saying they were perhaps the best side of all time. After all, they'd gone 24–1 through the 2000 season, including a 20-game winning streak, and had won their three finals by an aggregate 230 points, with a 10-goal win over Melbourne in the grand final. The Bombers were the benchmark, no doubt about it. Yet we beat them by 28 points at the Gabba in Round 10 and would beat them again, by 26 points, on grand final day at the MCG. And that was after we'd had a mixed 4–3 start to the year heading into the history-changing game against Carlton in Round 8.

Leading into the 2001 season I'd stood down after four years as co-captain, allowing Michael Voss to do the job solo. I'd considered doing this 12 months earlier but was talked out of it by my old mate and Lions assistant coach Matty Armstrong. But there's no doubt it was the right thing to do.

There were two reasons. One, I was still having trouble doing all the training and I didn't feel comfortable being captain of the club and not being able to do a lot of what my teammates were doing. And there was no guarantee, too, that I wouldn't be on and off the ground again, as had become something of a regular thing. Two, I didn't really believe on principle in the concept of co-captains.

Make no mistake — when Vossy and I were appointed to do the job together, going into the 1997 season, it was right. Neither of us needed the job in our own right and it made good sense to share it. But that time had well and truly passed.

So I went and saw the coach. At first he was reluctant to accept my decision, but he agreed to think about it. He came back to me a couple of days later with a compromise — he would accept it on the basis that I'd act and play the same as I'd always done. I was happy with that. You always want to give your utmost in a leadership sense anyway; it was more the title I didn't feel comfortable with. So I continued as almost an associate member of the leadership group which in 2001 saw Justin Leppitsch, Chris Scott, Nigel Lappin and Darryl White as understudies to Vossy. I was involved in all the leadership group meetings and did everything I'd previously done, but we had one captain. That was very important. And the fact that our peers in the AFL Players' Association voted Vossy Best Captain in 2001, 2002, 2003 and 2004 proved that it was the right decision.

It was all a bit of a fairytale. Things fell into place at the right time in 2001. We didn't have too many injury disruptions and got to grand final day with a full complement of senior players available. That is a critical component of any premiership campaign. There's rarely much difference between the sides, which means that any side can win the flag if most things are going pretty well right. That makes Port Adelaide's win in 2004 all the more impressive — they did it without All-Australian players Matthew Primus and Josh Francou.

It's so much about being in the right place at the right time. Just ask Mal Michael and Martin Pike. In 2000 big Mal had played his fourth season at Collingwood, but when Jarrod Molloy, a one-time Fitzroy player then at Brisbane, expressed his desire to go back to Melbourne and to join Collingwood, Magpies coach Mick Malthouse happily agreed to trade Molloy for the former Queenslander, who had done a couple of pre-season campaigns with the Bears in my early days in Brisbane. Across town Pikey had played his fourth season at North Melbourne, but despite having been a member of the Kangaroos' 1999 premiership side, he was de-listed by Denis Pagan. That wasn't so much a football decision as a personal one. Pikey had a perceived colourful off-field record and Pagan decided he'd had enough. So Leigh Matthews pounced. After consulting with some senior players he threw the veteran utility/defender a lifeline. He chose him with selection No. 33 in the 2000 national draft.

Bit by bit the puzzle was coming together. We already had a quality-plus midfield, with the likes of Michael Voss, Nigel Lappin, Jason Akermanis and an emerging Simon Black, plus Justin Leppitsch as the cornerstone of our defensive group. Now we had a proven fullback in Mal Michael and a cagey utility type, Martin Pike, who could be used as a pinch-hitter just about anywhere and would bolster our big-time experience.

There was one key component missing. It was the most important position on the field: centre half forward. But I knew we had it covered. Jonathan Brown was only 19 going into the 2001 season, but already he'd stamped himself as a star in the making. During the 1999–2000 pre-season I'd done some one-on-one marking work with him and I was amazed by his strength. Not so much by his actual strength, although that was there. It was more the way he knew how to use it. For a teenager, he had a lot of smarts. Guess that's what you get when you come from the bush. And he had a great aerobic capacity, too. He could run all day. It was a pretty awesome package.

After the all-important win over Essendon, we beat West Coast by 22 points in Perth, followed by Melbourne, Hawthorn and St Kilda at the Gabba. And by handy margins — 49 points, 87 points and 57 points. Then Collingwood at the MCG by 26 points. That was an important win, because it was our only home-and-away visit to headquarters for the year. Then Port Adelaide at the Gabba by 34 points, at which point we were second on the ladder, behind Essendon. Then North Melbourne at Colonial Stadium by 21 points, the Western Bulldogs by 33 points at the Gabba and Richmond by 31 points at the Gabba. It was 10 in a row. The same number of wins we'd strung together in 1999 before falling in the preliminary final.

In Round 20, 2001, I made what would be my last trip to Perth. Whether or not I'd go had been a contentious matter for some time. There was a growing suspicion that long-distance travel and CFS didn't go well together and the supporting evidence was mounting. In 1999 I hadn't put it to the test. The Lions travelled west twice in the first five rounds, when I wasn't playing. In Round 7, 2000, I went goal-less against Fremantle on Anzac Day and didn't play the following week. And in Round 11, 2001, I'd kicked two goals against West Coast but pulled up more than a little dusty. The eight goals I kicked the following week against Melbourne at the Gabba were as ordinary as eight-goal contributions come. I was lucky. Things just fell my way — eight times.

I shouldn't have played. I nearly didn't. Only the efforts of Alan Jansson got me over the line. He practised Japanese acupuncture. I'd been introduced to him through club physiotherapist Victor Popov, and he'd become a critical ally and a key part of my medical protocol. His treatment really helped my post-game recovery and I was seeing him once — often twice — a week at his clinic at Chandler.

I'd seen Alan twice in the week after our visit to Perth, but early on the Sunday morning of the Round 12 game against the Demons at the Gabba I was still struggling. Really struggling. I rang him at his Gold Coast home and told him I was about to call the coach and explain that I couldn't play. He advised me to wait. Without hesitating, he offered to drive up to Brisbane and treat me. Not just at his clinic. He came all the way to my home at Chapel Hill. He was there within 75 minutes. A few hours later I had one of those days and I kicked my eight goals. In the end, that probably swayed the argument in Round 20, so I returned to Perth for the game against Fremantle, but it was a touch and go call. And when I couldn't play the following week, in the 43-point Round 21 win over Geelong at Shell Stadium, that was it. The decision was made. Perth trips were off my schedule.

At least I would be spared an embarrassing repeat of one of my last trips to Perth when I flew with an oxygen tank for company. This was no two-hour flight to Melbourne so I did a series of 15-minute sessions on the bottle, breathing pure oxygen in the hope that it might help limit the detrimental impact of the longer period under cabin pressure conditions. It reduced my heart-rate by 10 per cent when on the oxygen at altitude but it didn't make any noticeable difference otherwise, and it was embarrassing when a hostess asked me if I needed a wheelchair to get me off the plane.

A Round 22 victory over Sydney by 31 points at the Gabba meant we'd won 13 in a row by an average margin of almost 40 points. But still we couldn't catch Essendon. We both had a 17–5 win/loss record, but the Bombers took the minor premiership on percentage.

Then came one of the scariest moments of my footy career. We beat third-placed Port Adelaide by 32 points at the Gabba in the qualifying final but I was reported on a striking charge. It was frightening. One week would be bad enough: I'd miss the preliminary final. But if I got two weeks I could miss playing in a grand final. I can't begin to describe what went through my mind. 'You idiot' was one thought.

Ordinarily I wouldn't make an extra trip to Melbourne, but I wasn't playing the following week regardless because we had the weekend off, so I headed south for the tribunal hearing instead of doing it via video-link from Brisbane. We just felt it was better for me to be there in person. Then I could look the tribunal members in the eye and exhibit genuine remorse for what had happened. It shouldn't have mattered, because there's no changing the video evidence, but it might have. Particularly when it came to sentencing. Whatever, we weren't about to take any chances.

Then came a huge shock. I was on my way to Melbourne when I was told that the club had decided to call Robert Walls as a character witness. At first I didn't like the idea. Not because I doubted his standing in the football world — he was among the most respected media commentators in the game and had had an outstanding career as a player and a coach. I just felt that he wasn't a fan of mine, and with a possible grand final appearance on the line I didn't want to take any chances.

I needn't have worried. Andrew Ireland, the Lions chief executive, and Gubby Allan, our football manager, convinced me it was a smart move because Wallsy wouldn't be seen as my all-time best mate jumping to my defence. If they'd wanted someone really close to me they would have called one of my former Fitzroy teammates to offer a character reference. Someone like Paul Roos.

Booked by a goal umpire on video evidence which showed me push Darryl Wakelin in the face with an open hand, I pleaded not guilty. I didn't think there was a lot in it. But after 90 minutes I was found guilty. I was going to get at least a week.

After the guilty verdict the club was allowed to speak in relation to penalty, as is normal procedure. Wallsy was fantastic, and after taking into account the fact that I'd never been suspended for striking in 14 years and 248 games and was the retaliator in the incident, the tribunal let me off with one week. I was out of there in double-quick time, knowing that the possibility of a grand final appearance now rested with my teammates.

Calling Wallsy as a witness was the making of our relationship. Or the restoring of a relationship which had started out very well when I moved to Brisbane in late 1993. As it turned out, I might have exaggerated things in my mind, and a very small crack between us had unreasonably become bigger. It's amazing how often that sort of thing can happen. You really are much better confronting an issue, even the smallest issue — you may well discover that it's not really an issue at all. Since then we've been very good friends. We'll always share a chat whenever we bump into each other, and he's been very generous in his support and the assistance he has offered me in many different ways.

I flew home from Melbourne straight after the tribunal and flicked on the television to catch the late news. I couldn't believe my eyes. A plane had just crashed into a World Trade Center tower in New York. And then, in front of my very eyes, another plane crashed into the adjacent tower. Thousands of people were dying. What a reality check. What a way to put things in perspective. All of a sudden my one-match suspension wasn't important. And there I sat, like most of the world, until about 5am, unable to switch off the television.

I might not have played in the preliminary final even if I'd not been suspended. In the first final I'd copped a whack in the back which had caused an old stress fracture to flare up. There was a lot of nerve irritation because of an unstable vertebra, and as it turned out I needed every hour of the three weeks between the qualifying final and the grand final to get myself into reasonable shape.

Still, watching the preliminary final against Richmond was one of the toughest things I've done. I felt bad that I wasn't able to contribute, and fearful that, having come so far, I might be denied one last chance to take that final step.

The boys put my mind at rest early. We led by 38 points at half-time and 60 points at three-quarter time, and I enjoyed the final quarter enormously. It wasn't quite in line with Leigh Matthews' formula — you're not safe until the number of goals you're ahead is more than the number of minutes left — but 10 goals at the last change was good enough for me.

There was excitement in the rooms after the win. After all, it's not every day you qualify for your first grand final. But it wasn't anything over the top. That was a good sign, because there was still so much to do. And all of a sudden we were in uncharted waters. Martin Pike aside, none of the Lions players had played in a flag decider, but we did have a certain coach who knew a little bit about winning premierships.

Upstairs in the stands, Peta was going through an altogether different set of emotions. She had sat through the preliminary final with Sharlene Broderick, who was nursing her new-born baby Lily (her two-year-old son Josh was in the Lions' crèche). My good mate Paul Broderick was playing for Richmond, so the girls watched the game knowing that one of their husbands would be in a grand final the following week and the other would be shattered. But the Tigers' loss actually meant more to 'Porky'. Not only did he not get to play in a grand final; it was also his last game. A sad end to the great career of a great mate.

Grand final week. It was a week like nothing I'd ever experienced. There was so much more than just football to worry about. On the Sunday afternoon, immediately after the normal recovery session, Leigh called a meeting with wives and girlfriends to outline the procedural matters. It was important to get on top of these things early — we couldn't let them become distractions. Things like flights, tickets, accommodation. That Ansett, the official AFL airline, had collapsed not long before only added to the task. We had to charter two 91-seat Flight West jets to transport everyone connected with the club to Melbourne on the Thursday. In what was a total contrast to normal procedure, the girls and kids travelled with the players. So, too, did non-football management, directors, and even some sponsors and supporters. Ordinarily the coach's instruction was to keep things as normal as possible, but there was no alternative this time.

And as it turned out, it was a blessing. Because we had the plane to ourselves, we could do as we wished. There were no flight attendants telling us to sit down, and no other passengers to consider. Having a lot of kids there helped ease the tension, too — although none of them were mine. Peta took Madison and our new son, Tom, to Melbourne earlier in the week. We'd talked about what the best approach would be for us all, and that was what we had come up with. She'd filled the fridge with food and left me to focus on getting fit and ready for the day I'd waited all my life for.

It was a busy week. Monday was a media free-for-all. It was good to get the bulk of that out of the way. Tuesday was the normal review meeting. Wednesday we trained at Coorparoo in front of a huge crowd. Thursday we were off to Melbourne. On top of this, I had twice daily sessions with physiotherapist Peter Stanton. My fate was in his hands, literally. 'Stants' is the most thorough medical practitioner I know. He left nothing to chance, except perhaps the timing of his next appointment — he was rarely on time, because he would work right through a problem to the very end. And this week I really needed it.

Leigh Matthews had encouraged the players to 'live in a bubble' during grand final week, to observe and enjoy all the things going on around us, but not to let them penetrate our psyche or become a distraction. It was good advice, but it wasn't quite as simple as that for Jason Akermanis, who had won the Brownlow Medal on the Monday night. With that came extra pressures and responsibilities, but 'Aka' took it all in his stride, as he does, and just tried to focus on the game.

We stayed where we always stayed in Melbourne: in the Park View Hotel on St Kilda Road. We'd been going there for three years and it was like our second home. Everything there was now so normal and familiar. By the time we arrived on Thursday evening it was basically dinner, a catch-up coffee with Peta, who I hadn't seen for three days, another session with Stants and bed.

Friday morning was more physio and then the Grand Final Parade through the streets of Melbourne. I'd heard stories about how the parade could be a bit of a chore, but I loved it. All of us planned to enjoy it. We'd worked so hard for so long to get to this point, so why not? I took Madison in the parade with me, which was great. The crowd support was incredible. It was a mass of maroon, blue and gold. The Fitzroy faithful and the multitudes who had travelled from Brisbane via any and every means of transport available easily outnumbered the Essendon supporters among the crowd of 100,000-plus.

On Friday afternoon we had a short, low-intensity training session at Albert Cricket Ground, opposite the team hotel. There was a huge crowd again. Then it was the usual team meeting, where Leigh Matthews outlined the team and a few specific individual roles, and identified a couple of things we would try to do to exploit the opposition structure. His message was simple — do what you always do. Stick to the game plan and the team principles. The meeting didn't last more than an hour and then it was time for dinner, a bit of a chat among the boys, another quick session with Stants and off to bed. I took a sleeping tablet and, surprisingly, I had a pretty good sleep.

I'm not normally a nervous person, and during the week my focus had been on the countless hours with Stants trying to get my back right. This was probably a good thing, because it helped keep my mind off other things. The group in general, too, was usually pretty confident and chirpy, and breakfast on match days was full of chat and jokes. Not grand final day. There were 20-odd players there when I ate, and all you could hear was knives and forks. I couldn't help myself — I said 'Is anyone nervous?' That broke the ice a little, but it was so quiet. Nobody quite knew what to say. We were within hours of fulfilling a lifetime dream and there was no textbook on how you were supposed to act.

I got a fantastic surprise after breakfast when the hotel reception sent a good luck card up to my room. It was from Peta. She'd walked all the way from the Holiday Inn, where the girls were staying, to deliver it at about 8am. She was rooming with Rosanne Bayes, wife of our runner and ex-Swans champion Mark Bayes, and Lisa O'Donnell, wife of assistant coach and ex-Essendon captain Gary O'Donnell, and had gone for a leisurely 10km stroll with Lisa on grand final morning. It was a really nice gesture, and something she'd repeat each of the next three years with Lisa, Rosanne and Donna Voss. Pete, whose sister Claire was looking after Madison and Tom, has a happy knack of finding just the right words. She didn't stay, even to say hello, because she didn't want to be a distraction; her only disappointment was being nabbed by the Channel Seven cameras as she left the hotel. She doesn't like publicity, preferring to stay completely out of the public eye.

At midday the team bus left the hotel under police escort for the trip to the MCG. At 12.30pm, after the end of the early game, we had a chance to walk down the race from our dressing rooms under the old Olympic Stand and out onto the ground for the pre-game warm-up. It was earlier than normal because of the pre-game entertainment, but it didn't matter. This wasn't about warming up. We'd do that thoroughly in the rooms later. This was about the moment. There were already 60,000 people inside this fabulous arena and it was an important time. We didn't play too often at the 'G' — only once previously in 2001 and twice (including a semi-final) in 2000 — so it was good to get a feel for it. It really helped ease the tension among the group and remove the temptation to think that grand final day was going to be any different from a normal game. Sure, the stakes were as high as they could possibly get, but it was still a game of football. We weren't going to a mystical place that we'd never been to before, despite that being how the MCG on grand final day is sometimes portrayed.

I don't remember too many specific details of the next hour and a half. It was business as usual. Strapping, massage and special medical treatment. Each player had his own routine. The coach spoke to the players at 1pm and he played a five-minute motivational videotape which we'd also seen the night before. Put to the music of 'Dare to Dream', sung by Olivia Newton-John and John Farnham at the 2000 Sydney Olympics, it highlighted extra special efforts of each player during the finals. It wasn't big marks and big goals; it was the little things, like tackles and spoils. The team things. It wasn't supposed to have players jumping around the room, with the hair on the back of their neck standing on end 90 minutes before game time, but the message was clear and simple. Together we would win. We would be doing it for each other.

Relying on each other. Just as we'd done since that afternoon at Optus Oval in Round 8. It didn't matter how many times Leigh Matthews had said it — he had the ability to make sure it never sounded repetitive.

I remember walking down the race for the game. The moment somebody opened the dressing room door the noise filtered up into the rooms, but as we hit the ground the roar was deafening. My feet felt like they didn't hit the ground for the first 30m of the customary stride-through. I'd always been last onto the ground as a kid, but I'd long since surrendered that right. It must be a kid thing, because now Jonathan Brown, who was just 19, was always last out.

Michael Voss went to the middle of the ground to toss the coin and I gathered the players together. I'm not sure if anyone was listening or taking too much notice, but I reiterated what had been the message from the coach all year. Don't worry about anything except your role in the team. Don't worry about the result. It had been said often during the week and had helped ease the nerves a lot, because this way it wasn't Brisbane trying to beat the might of Essendon — it was 22 players being predictable to their teammates.

The grand final wasn't too old when I copped a high whack from Bombers fullback Dustin Fletcher which I later learned had perforated my eardrum. It wasn't as serious as it might sound, but it made sure the loud roar of the crowd was more like a dull drone for the rest of the day. I lined up a free kick from about 35m and tried to go through my normal routine. I've not got what you'd call a classical kicking style and I've always felt most comfortable if I talk to myself as I go back. 'It's the first shot at goal in a grand final — don't miss it,' I said. So what did I do? I pulled it left. Happily, a couple of minutes later I got another free kick for a high tackle by John Barnes and managed to steer that one through. We were away.

At quarter-time we led by five points, but it could and should have been more. It was 3.7 to 3.2. We'd missed a few opportunities. And when the Bombers got five of the first six goals of the second term we were 20 points down. At the 33-minute mark, Simon Black turned his opponent inside out and, on his non-preferred right foot, hit me on the chest lace out. It was an important one, and though it might not have come off the boot perfectly, it sailed through from 40m. We'd been outscored by 19 points for the quarter and were 14 points down: 5.10 to 8.6.

Still, it was the most relaxed I'd ever seen our team when we were behind at half-time. Everyone just went about their business as usual. It was one of the hottest grand finals in a long time and most players spent some time in the cool room. This had been set up in the sauna to help lower the core body temperature after the AFL had banned the club's use of intravenous drips as a half-time means of rehydration.

It wasn't anything new — we'd been doing it for a couple of years — but after the qualifying final win over Port Adelaide the story had broken in the media and the AFL felt obliged to act.

I thought that was wrong because it was totally legal and was nothing more than expert medical practitioners doing their utmost to aid the recovery of their patients, which, after all, is exactly what they are supposed to do. It was only ever done under the most hygienic conditions, and reports of players having shunts in their arm, so they could insert the drip quickly at half-time were just ridiculous.

The club had got right on the front foot over the IV drip issue, rightfully supporting the medical team, but I could also see the AFL viewpoint. The mental picture of players en masse sitting around at half-time with drips in their arms wasn't a good one. And as much as what we do has no direct correlation with what others do, we always have to be mindful of our responsibilities as role models to the kids.

But by half-time on grand final day it was a non-issue.
I've got no idea what the coach said; it didn't matter. You
could just tell there was an air of confidence among the
group. We'd wasted a few opportunities, but within ourselves
we knew that if we just kept doing what we'd been doing for
most of the year, things would turn around. We had a steely
belief in each other. After all, we'd won 15 in a row, and we
were very confident we'd be able to outrun the opposition in
the second half. And that's exactly what happened. The
ability of the midfielders to keep running was just incredible.

By three-quarter time we led by 16 points, having
kicked 6.2 to 1.2 for the term. It was all going to come
down to the last quarter. Our 100th quarter for the season.
Matthew Lloyd got the first goal for Essendon, but Tim
Notting helicoptered one through for us and then Beau
McDonald took the ball out of a boundary throw-in and
fed Michael Voss for another. We were 16 minutes in and
26 points up. You could sense the excitement building.
Luke Power and Jason Akermanis made sure of it.

I remembered John Blakey, a premiership player with
the Kangaroos in 1996 and 1999, saying to me that the
sweetest moment in football is when you're playing a
grand final and you know you've got it won. But Essendon
kicked a couple of quick ones to keep it alive. I felt we

couldn't relax until the final siren went. It was as good as it gets for a boy from north-west Tasmania who used to dream of kicking the winning goal in an AFL grand final or opening the bowling for the Australian cricket team and didn't really think either was any chance.

It was one big celebration from that moment on. The presentations, the photographs, the lap of honour and the team-only moment in the coach's room. Sharing the moment with family and friends in the changing rooms was special, too. Untold hugs, handshakes and back slaps in between umpteen thousand photographs. Everyone wanted a shot with the premiership cup. And everyone got one. A team photo with the cup in the semi-darkness right in the centre circle of the MCG was one to keep.

Finally, about two hours later, the team bus pulled out of the MCG. It might have been licensed to carry 50 passengers, but there must have been 100-plus. Nobody cared. Not even Senior Sergeant Hart, who was assigned to make sure we got where we were going. How appropriate: Shaun Hart had won the Norm Smith Medal and now his namesake, no relation, was the official protector of the premiership team.

Most players were so caught up in the emotion that even after they'd showered and dressed in the casual uniform of slacks and polo shirt, they put their dirty jumper back on over the top. With their premiership medals around their necks, of course. I couldn't bring myself to do it. My jumper smelt something terrible.

I sat in the front seat next to the coach, with the cup. It was a special moment, and something I would repeat every year after the grand final. There I was, with the coach, who was now only the second person in football history to win a premiership at three different clubs. Ron Barassi had done it with Melbourne, Carlton and North Melbourne, and now Leigh Matthews had done it with Hawthorn, Collingwood and the Brisbane Lions.

First stop was Rod Laver Arena at the Melbourne Tennis Centre, where about 5000 fans had been waiting for nearly three hours to salute the players. It was like a rock concert as we walked up onto the stage for interviews and, of course, a trademark Jason Akermanis handstand. And autographs. Heaps of them.

Then it was back to the team hotel briefly to drop off our bags, then straight back on the bus and off to Crown Casino, where 1600 corporate guests awaited us in the Palladium Ballroom for the official premiership dinner. Speeches, more handshakes, a few silly stories. The night had it all, including Dad, Mum and her partner Peter, and my brother Manuel and his wife Leonie. I didn't drink a lot because I wanted to savour the moment. And despite the excitement and euphoria, my CFS was still in the back of my mind. No point being silly. Finally Peta and I escaped with Mark and Rosanne Bayes to a private room downstairs, where we had a quiet coffee. The taxi queue was as long as the MCG, but just as we were about to begin walking to the hotel, Cathy Oswald, the Lions marketing manager, spotted us and redirected a car which had been driving some corporate guests. At about 3am I crashed for one of the most contented nights' sleep I'd had. Even if it lasted only a few hours.

The team bus left the hotel at 9am Sunday for the old Brunswick Street Oval, where 8000 fans were gathered. It was great to see a lot of familiar faces. The tears and the sheer joy said it all. It was good for the players, especially the younger ones, to see just how much it meant to the supporters. The raw emotion was incredible. Martin Pike, who had won the 1996 Fitzroy best and fairest before being overlooked in the original merger draft, managed to get hold of the microphone and pay special tribute to the unity of the Brisbane and Fitzroy supporter groups. And he offered a little free advice for those Fitzroy fans who had chosen not to support the merger.

On the flight home to Brisbane the pilot was given special clearance for a Gabba flyover. He came in low and dipped the wing over the ground, and out my side of the plane we looked straight down on the ground to see another 8000 people awaiting us for the next part of the celebration. It felt as if we almost flew in between the light towers — for a one-time nervous flyer like me it was a bit of a shocker.

The plan was for Peta to drop me off at the Gabba for another session with the fans and head home with the kids, but it didn't quite work out that way. Something had to go wrong in this glorious time, and it did: I'd managed to leave the car keys in the hotel room in Melbourne, and by the time the RACQ people got us going and we drove to the Gabba, the fans had gone. So it was just a BBQ and a few Crown Lagers for the inner-sanctum of the club.

On the Monday morning Peta dropped me off at the Australian National Hotel — the Aussie Nash — opposite the Gabba, for the traditional Mad Monday celebrations. They were sweeter than ever before, but I made a serious tactical error. It was only in the taxi on the way home a little after midnight that I realised the date. Monday had been 1 October. My wedding anniversary. I got the cabbie to pull into the BP petrol station at Kenmore and I grabbed two bunches of flowers. It had been a big day, and it was not until the following morning, when the haze started to wear off, that I realised the flowers I bought were plastic! No wonder they didn't go down as well as I'd hoped. Mind you, I have to say Pete was pretty good-humoured about it . . . however, she has reminded me a few times of the day I missed our wedding anniversary. Never again. Well, maybe just once more — in 2002.

There was no end in sight to the celebrations. On Tuesday a massive crowd turned out for a ticker-tape parade through the inner-city streets of Brisbane. In a supposedly non-AFL city it was extraordinary. I took Madison in the open-top car with me and she had a ball. It was a coming of age for AFL football in Queensland and I had a feeling that, regardless of their traditional football loyalties, people here now had a genuine soft spot for the Lions. It also made me realise how fortunate the Brisbane Lions were to genuinely be a two-town team. We had a strong and vibrant supporter base in Brisbane, and another in Melbourne. That was a real treat, and it was important in that it meant the only real away games we played were in Sydney, Adelaide and Perth.

Wednesday was lunch with Queensland Premier Peter Beattie and a bunch of top-level sponsors at Tattersall's

Club. Half an hour before we sat down, marketing manager Cathy Oswald told me Michael Voss couldn't make it because his wife Donna was ill. She is a diabetic, and had been rushed to hospital the day before. She was all right, but Vossy wasn't about to leave her. So I was thrust into the role of team spokesman.

We had a great story to tell. I spoke about grand final week, how we handled it and what it meant to the players. None of us should ever take things like the opportunity of winning a premiership for granted — you never know what is around the corner and whether it will come around again.

11

BELIEVE IT OR NOT

I was never much of a drinker as an AFL footballer. Certainly not in the last 12 years of my career. When I was out with teammates on a special end-of-season occasion there tended to be a lot of drunken pot plants — I'd look as if I was getting into the spirit of things, literally, but I'd sneakily pour most of the drinks out. It was the only way I could enjoy the occasion and look after myself at the same time. But in 2003 I found an unlikely ally in my endless battle with sleeping problems: alcohol.

Not beer or wine. I turned to Baileys or even an occasional vodka. During the season it was not unusual for me to drink a good portion of a bottle in one night early in a football week when I just couldn't get to sleep. It was the only thing that helped.

I'd shared in two AFL premierships by this stage, and was playing some of the best football of my career, but I was still having shocking problems with sleep. Sleep deprivation is a big part of the CFS story, but the extent of my trouble was kept secret. There was nothing to be gained by going public. And besides, I didn't want anyone knowing what I was doing to alleviate the problem — alcohol wasn't a good fit for an AFL footballer.

For a long time the only person who knew what was going on was my occasional night-time drinking partner, Peta. I even made sure I bought the Baileys from different places so that nobody would cotton on. You'd be surprised how many bottle shops there are between the Gabba and the western suburbs of Brisbane.

My sleep problem, especially early in the week, was two-fold. I struggled to get to sleep, and when I did sleep I didn't get enough quality sleep. If we played on a Saturday night I knew I'd never get to sleep that night. Often Sunday night would be spent in front of the television, too. So I'd be back at the club on the Monday feeling awful. Monday was usually only a massage day and perhaps a light jog, but my head would feel terrible and I'd have next to no energy. Not surprising, really, as I had been awake for going on 72 hours. And besides being bad for my football, it made simple things like driving a car dangerous. Not a good situation.

The more tired I got, the harder it was for me to get to sleep. The more I didn't sleep, the more I couldn't sleep. It sounds backwards, but that's the way it worked. The only sleep I could ever manage early in the week was really shallow sleep that didn't provide any quality physical recovery. I couldn't get into what is called REM sleep. Rapid eye movement sleep, or stage four sleep, is when your body really recharges itself. And because I'd used sleeping tablets so often over the years I was pretty much immune to them. None of them would work.

One day I thought I'd try a couple of beers. They helped me get off to sleep all right but I woke up feeling a bit sluggish. Having had virtually no alcohol since the onset of my CFS, my system didn't handle it well. So beer was out. Likewise wine. It had the same effect. Initially, vodka was doing the job nicely until one night I had a Baileys and it worked just as well — and it was probably a bit easier to drink.

I didn't discuss it with anyone because I knew what people would say. And it was a bit embarrassing, too —

Baileys isn't the most masculine drink. Eventually, I dropped it into conversation with a couple of teammates at training. Jonathan Brown had a big laugh but by then I didn't care so much. It worked when all else failed, so I turned to it for occasional help.

In retirement I've shared this story with a few more people and they've all been blown away. They couldn't believe that even in 2003 I was still having major problems.

Now, I'm a light social drinker — an occasional beer or a glass of wine with a meal, and a few beers with the boys at tennis on Wednesday nights.

Meanwhile, I was having trouble believing the remarkable story of the Brisbane Lions. I don't think the 2001 grand final win really sank in until I was on holidays at Mooloolaba on Queensland's Sunshine Coast. My family had a fantastic three-week break there, and it was only then, away from the normal football environment, that I had time to reflect on it. I'd be playing with the kids on the beach and strangers would come up and say, 'I just wanted to say congratulations — what the Lions have been able to do is just fantastic.' They didn't intrude or impose, but were genuinely touched by what was a real football fairytale. I loved that, and really appreciated it.

One premiership was hard to comprehend. Two was even more difficult, and three in a row was almost impossible. Even a couple of years on, I still find it quite extraordinary that I was part of such an incredible success story.

I blame Leigh Matthews for this. Or I should say, I credit Leigh Matthews. One of his strongest messages to the playing group in the wake of the 2001 premiership was that we should simply live in the moment. Not worry about what was in the past or what was in the future, just focus on the task at hand.

In 2002 we didn't set out to win back-to-back premierships — we were only trying to win one premiership. It just so happened that if we were successful it would give us two in a row. Sounds simple, I know, but it was true.

I remember the first day back at training in November 2001. It still seemed a bit unreal, sitting in the team meeting knowing that we were all premiership winners, but what really struck me when we got down to the hard grind of pre-season training was that the players were able to focus just as they had done 12 months earlier. There was no premiership hangover. Everyone was just going about their business as normal, driven by a desire to make themselves better. They knew that by doing that, by fulfilling their individual roles at a higher level than the previous year, they could make the team better.

There was intense competition within the group, which was a healthy thing. The attention was on everything but the 2002 grand final. It was, for each individual, about putting themselves in a better physical position than 12 months before. Which of the big boys would lift the most weight in the gym? Perhaps Mal Michael, Daniel Bradshaw, a young Jonathan Brown or the Scott twins? Would anyone threaten Shaun Hart or Simon Black for the endurance running crown? Who might challenge Brad Scott and Jason Akermanis over 20m? The strength of mind of the playing group was really sensational, and long before season 2002 got under way I knew we were going to be right in the mix again.

Personally, I had a quiet summer. And not just because I didn't want to tempt CFS in the hot weather. I had an Achilles problem which I'd carried through much of the 2001 campaign and it wouldn't allow me to do anything much more than swim, ride the bike and push a few weights in the gym. Health management was my priority.

We didn't talk about back-to-back premierships but one person did: Malcolm Blight, the 1978 Brownlow medallist and Adelaide Crows coach during their consecutive premiership years of 1997 and 1998. Leigh Matthews asked him to address our group about the mindset of defending the crown and he said much the same things as our own coach. Blight had, of course, been lured back into coaching in 2001 by St Kilda, only to be sacked in sensational fashion two-thirds of the way through the year. As he walked into the Gabba meeting room and saw the complicated mix of words and diagrams on the whiteboard he said, 'If only I'd known that a couple of years ago.' Then he won an even bigger laugh when he said: 'The last time I was in a situation like this, talking to a group of AFL footballers, I said, "See you tomorrow" and I didn't.'

The other big issue of the 2001–02 summer was pay cuts. Not long after the 2001 premiership, the playing group was advised in no uncertain terms that the club wouldn't be able to keep the entire group together unless some players were prepared to make a sacrifice. Or, as Leigh Matthews preferred to put it, to invest in the group in the interests of being part of a successful team.

In four years we'd experienced the extremes of AFL football — a wooden spoon in 1998 and a premiership in 2001. And there was no way anyone wanted to go back to the days of '98 when football wasn't fun and it was a chore just to go to the club for training.

I wasn't one of the players asked to take a pay cut because I wasn't in the top pay bracket. By 2002, football inflation had caught up with my 10-year contract and put me in the mid-range category. Not that I had any gripes. The security of my contract had been fantastic and I fully understood and accepted that others were now being paid more.

Much was made of the pay cuts in the media but the players didn't see it as a big deal. Leigh brought me into the discussions so I was aware of what was going on: the players were eager to do whatever it took to keep the group together.

We were very tight. A premiership does that to a playing group. And the opportunity to chase a second flag made us even tighter. The prospect of losing a quality member of the group, both from a personal and football viewpoint, wasn't something the players would entertain.

You don't measure your career by how much money you make. To even suggest that is ludicrous. You measure your career by team success and friendships, because they are the two things you remember most. Even individual honours, as satisfying as they are, rate well back in priority compared with premierships and people.

So about a dozen players made a quick and easy decision to do what was required to keep the group together and we moved on. It wasn't spoken about again. At not least within my earshot.

We won the first four games of 2002, which stretched our winning streak to 20. It was the equal second-longest streak in history. Only Geelong's 23-game stretch in 1952–53 was better. This made the decision for me not to travel to Perth for the Round 5 game against West Coast very difficult. The temptation to go and perhaps help keep the streak alive was huge, but Leigh Matthews put his foot down. We'd made a decision about this, because we knew that long travel wasn't good for me, and after ignoring our own rule a couple of times and paying the price, he wasn't about to waver. It was no fun watching the game on television and seeing us go down to the Eagles by 46 points, but I knew that I wouldn't have made the difference. And when I kicked five goals the following week against Geelong at the Gabba, we knew we'd made the right decision.

In Round 14 another streak ended. After 18 consecutive Gabba wins, dating back to the start of the premiership push in Round 10, 2001, we lost there to Melbourne. It was an odd game. We kicked 8.3 to 2.2 in the first quarter and still led by 39 points early in the third quarter, but then were overrun by the Demons and lost by 21 points.

It was like the annual wake-up call we had to have. It was the first time we'd conceded 20 goals in a game since Round 8 against Carlton at Optus Oval in 2001, and just as that defeat had jolted us into action, this would do likewise. It served as a reminder of the team-first and role-playing ethos which had been the keystone of our success. Getting flash and individualistic was never going to work. We had to stick to the plan.

I was an immediate beneficiary, kicking back-to-back bags of seven goals in the next two weeks. It's amazing what a difference it makes at full forward when your side gets the ball in quickly. This was the beginning of a small winning streak: seven games, and an average margin of eight goals. We were in good touch, but we still went into Round 22 against Port Adelaide at Football Park needing to win to clinch the minor premiership.

The halfway point of the seven-win streak was one of football's more memorable games: the 'no rules' game. Essendon coach Kevin Sheedy had warned us in the lead-up, saying: 'If I was Brisbane, I wouldn't treat Essendon without respect, because our players will be pretty pumped up for this game. I will just tell the players there are no rules ... none whatsoever. Anything can happen, that's for sure.'

It did. We won by 37 points and 10 Lions and six Bombers, reported on a total of 17 charges, were fined a total of $14,400 and suspended for four matches. An accidental back-hander to Dustin Fletcher as I led for the ball cost me two weeks, but at least I managed to be at the right end of the ground to avoid the melee. After the $4000 fine against Richmond in 1998 and $3000 for pulling teammate Simon Black out of a melee against Essendon 16 weeks earlier, I didn't need another hit in the pocket on top of a two-week suspension.

Out of two Brisbane–Essendon games in 2002 the AFL picked up $31,600 in melee fines — all for 60 seconds' worth of pushing and shoving. Leigh Matthews suggested before the tribunal hearing for the 'no rules' game that they shouldn't penalise the players for putting on one of the best spectacles in a long time. I agreed with him. While I understand where the AFL was coming from, wanting to stamp out unsightly congregations of players, the fines were getting a little out of hand.

In Round 22 Leigh pulled a masterstroke. Though it was a huge game, with top spot and possibly a home preliminary final resting on the outcome, he recognised that irrespective of what happened, the following week was going to be bigger: it was going to be a final. So it was business as usual in our build-up. Port, in contrast, seemed to treat it like a final. When their players ran onto the ground their hair was wet and their eyes were spinning. They were really pumped. They were too good and won by six points, sure, we were disappointed but Port looked like they'd won the flag when the final siren went.

The Power paid the price six days later, suffering an awful letdown. They were beaten by fourth-placed Collingwood by 13 points at Football Park on the Friday night. This meant that when we played Adelaide, 24 hours later, we would claim the all-important home ground advantage for the preliminary final if we beat them. We did — by 71 points.

You hear it all the time — the finals are a new season — and it's absolutely right. You spend all year getting into the best position to launch a finals campaign and then you try to take things up a notch. After a week off, we beat a demoralised Port by 56 points in the preliminary final to qualify for our second consecutive grand final. This time it would be against Collingwood, who had timed their run perfectly through a fantastic finals series.

It was so different the second year, and yet so similar. We did virtually everything the same way we'd done it a year

earlier. We even picked up another Brownlow Medal via
Simon Black. But because we'd been through it all before,
the playing group was much more relaxed. Instead of
Martin Pike being the only premiership player in our side,
we had 20. The only changes from the 2001 premiership
side were that Des Headland and Aaron Shattock had
replaced Daniel Bradshaw and Robbie Copeland. The
message was the same: play your role, and don't worry
about anything else.

There were no suspension worries for me in 2002, but I
had another problem: a crook back, again. I played in the
grand final under painkilling injections. The medical staff,
my favourite people at this time of year, tested it at
training on the Friday night and got me through again on
the Saturday afternoon.

I might also have sent them to Hobart to look after
Dad. He was in hospital preparing for a quintuple heart
bypass. The surgery was scheduled for the Thursday after
the grand final, but what worried me most was the fact
that the surgeon was a Collingwood supporter! Obviously,
Dad didn't get over for the premiership decider.

If you're a full forward, the last thing you want to see
when you wake up on grand final day is bad weather. We
got it in trumps in 2002. It was bitterly cold, with driving

rain. Instead of the brilliant sunshine and 33°C that we enjoyed in 2001, the mercury struggled to reach double figures. It was no surprise, then, that the contest became a long, hard, physical slog. There were never more than nine points in it. And that was at the final siren.

I've always believed that betting on football is a mug's game, because there are too many unpredictables. And the most unpredictable game of the year is the grand final.

According to the papers, the television and the radio, it was going to be a no-contest. We were raging hot favourites, and Collingwood might just as well have stayed at home. They were no chance. But it was never going to be anything like that, especially when the wet weather set in.

The lead changed hands 13 times and scores were level four times. Eleven minutes into the final quarter, Magpies ruckman Josh Fraser put his side in front by three points.

I remember the next 16 or 17 minutes vividly. It was a bit like the next chapter in the fairytale of 2001. This was the one where I kicked the goal to get us back in front.

Two minutes after the Fraser goal Luke Power did brilliantly well to win possession at half forward and give a handpass to Michael Voss, who bombed it long to the square. I was taken out early by my opponent Shane Wakelin and received a free kick. This was the moment dreams are made of: a chance to kick what might have been the winning goal. I was 20m out on a slight angle. It should have been simple, but nothing was simple in this weather. All I focused on was making sure I got far enough back from the man on the mark, dropped the ball straight and kept my head over it so I'd kick through it. And yes, I did have my usual 'hope I don't miss'. But I managed to steer it through. We were three points up.

Scoring was difficult in those weather conditions, so it was 10 minutes before the next goal. Brad Scott gathered at centre half forward and bombed it in long to the hot spot. Moments earlier Jason Akermanis had got a message from the coach via runner Craig Starcevich to get to the front of me when the ball came in. He'd been running to the back, working on the principle that the wet, slippery ball might slip through, but Leigh was on the money. Shane Wakelin got a fist in to spoil and the ball came to the front. Aka was in just the right spot and found himself in space. 'You've got time,' I screamed loudly — it had to be loud if he was to hear it. He steadied and pulled it back over his right shoulder with his left foot. Goal. We were nine points up. There were six minutes still to play, but this was the last score of the grand final. We were home.

The emotion when the final siren went was totally different from the indescribable adrenaline rush and excitement of 2001. It was nothing but pure relief. Every player on both sides was exhausted. We were just fortunate to have finished in front. Now we were the sixth team since 1960 to win back-to-back flags.

We went through the presentation of the Norm Smith Medal to Collingwood captain Nathan Buckley and the individual premiership medallions. I can remember big Beau McDonald running over to the group just in time. He had socks on his feet and his shoulder in a sling, and he looked as if his eyes were spinning. He'd just come from hospital, and had been heavily sedated so doctors could repair a dislocation.

It hadn't been a good day for big 'Hat Rack'. He'd only been on the ground four minutes when he popped his shoulder at a boundary throw-in. Medical staff had been unable to get it back in at the ground, so off he went to hospital. Luckily, Alex Gardner, one of the army of volunteer helpers, went with him, because when they got back to the MCG in a taxi, Beau did a runner as the final siren sounded. Without any money, he left Alex to pay the cabbie. But Beau didn't care — he had a second premiership medallion.

Leigh Matthews had received the Jock McHale Medal from Graeme Reynolds, son of the late Dick Reynolds, former Essendon champion and triple Brownlow medallist, and was standing beside Michael Voss. They were about to receive the cup when Vossy screamed out to me to join him on the stage. I was a bit hesitant, but eventually that childhood dream took over and up I went to stand between the coach and the captain to receive the cup from Richmond 400-gamer Kevin Bartlett.

It all went back to a promise Vossy had made almost two years earlier, when I'd stepped down as co-captain. He'd said to me that if ever we won a flag he'd get me up to share the presentation with him. In the excitement of 2001 he forgot. So did I. And I hadn't given it a thought in 2002, either, until he screamed out to me. Another dream come true.

Initially the celebrations weren't quite as boisterous as the year before, but soon enough things got into full swing. We went through the full cycle again, and once more, it wasn't until I was up on the beach at Mooloolaba, accepting the congratulations from many of the same strangers, that it all sank in. Again. I'd been part of back-to-back premiership teams. I'd kicked a then career-best 74 goals in 22 games, including 16 in three finals — that was a personal bonus. I was proud of that, but in the big picture it didn't matter. Probably none of the people on the beach knew that or cared about it. But they all knew the Lions had won the flag. Again.

The big personnel change from 2002 to 2003 was the loss of Des Headland, a former No. 1 draft pick who had had a real roller-coaster ride in Brisbane: a goal with his first kick in League footy in 1999, 20 home-and-away games in 2001 before missing selection for all three finals, and then a starring role in the 2002 premiership campaign, when he kicked 34 goals in 20 games and stormed home to finish equal sixth in the Brownlow Medal count.

It wasn't a football decision. If it was, I have no doubt he would have stayed and been a very good player for the Lions for a long time. It was a family decision. Des and partner Chantelle had a one-year-old daughter, Madisan, and Chantelle's mother was keen for the young family to go home to Perth. So Des asked to be traded to one of the Perth-based clubs.

It was an issue which really tugged at the heartstrings of the Brisbane Lions, particularly Leigh Matthews, who had to make the final call. Essentially, Leigh was being asked to release a quality player on family grounds. To put Des's family ahead of the interests of the football club. He could have dug his heels in and forced Des into the draft as an out-of-contract player, possibly denying him the chance to move home and live with his family, and at the same time ensuring that the Lions received no compensation.

But eventually, after much public and private debate, Leigh decided he couldn't stand in the way of a young family. So the Lions accepted a trade which sent Des to the Fremantle Dockers, moved young Docker Adam McPhee to Essendon with young Lion Damian Cupido, and brought us Blake Caracella, an Essendon premiership player in 2000 and a member of the Bombers side we had beaten in the 2001 grand final.

It was no surprise, in hindsight, that Des was the last player off the ground after the 2002 grand final lap of honour. Having missed out in 2001, he was determined to enjoy every last second of it. Perhaps he knew he was leaving, despite public comments to the contrary in the days after the premiership was won.

Just as Des Headland left a tight-knit group in Brisbane, Blake Caracella had to try to break into one. Forced to leave Essendon by salary cap pressures, he chose Brisbane over Geelong, and then had to make it work. It couldn't have been easy. Football clubs are generally very welcoming places, but when a group of guys have been together for a long time and won two flags, they can be pretty set in their ways. It wouldn't have helped, either, leaving an equally close player group at Essendon, where he'd enjoyed premiership success. And Brisbane would have been seen as the enemy. Still, in the end Blake did it really well. He managed to create a niche for himself within the Lions group and become a popular and well-respected player.

Season 2003 was waged in three parts. We had eight wins and a draw in the first 10 rounds, lost six of the next 10 to slip to sixth on the ladder, and then the finals. Happily, that would bring further success.

I was feeling reasonably good by now, and we had the CFS under reasonable control, but every now and then it would send out a little reminder. Like in Round 1 against Essendon at the Gabba. My blood pressure dropped, I spent a lot of time off the ground and I was ill after the game. A couple of days later Leigh Matthews told me he wasn't taking me to Adelaide the following week to play Port Adelaide at Football Park. As the week wore on I started to feel better, and I told him, 'I'll be right — I want to play.' It was the only time I overruled the boss. Never again. I didn't last long, was really crook, and didn't play in Round 3, against the Kangaroos at the Telstra Dome.

Round 7 was a special day for the club. We played
Sydney at the SCG in Marcus Ashcroft's 300th game.
'Choppers' was the first Queenslander to post a triple
century, and the first player to reach that milestone who had
spent his entire career outside Victoria. It was a sensational
effort when you think how much he'd had to travel. He'd
survived the dark years at Carrara and seen the club grow
from a laughing stock to a benchmark. His absolute
professionalism and his attention to detail in his preparation
had seen him play 170 games in a row from 1992 to 2000.
He'd reinvented himself when Leigh Matthews came to the
club, switching to a no-frills role in defence after playing his
early days as a free-running midfielder-cum-forward. A
perfect example of a player who accepted a role within the
team structure, and just went out each week and did his job.
Sadly, we lost his 300th game by 19 points.

Our annual wake-up call came mid-year, as usual. In
Round 12, against West Coast at the Gabba. The Eagles
smashed us by 10 goals. It was the first time since the 2002
wake-up call from Melbourne that we'd conceded 20-plus
goals.

I remember the game most particularly because of the
way Chris Judd played. How quick was he? Incredible. He
had five goals at half-time and was sensational. It took me

back to a comment by Leigh Matthews when we played West Coast late in 2002. In the pre-game meeting he told us to ignore the fact that Judd was a first-year player because he was already a star, and a genuine match-winner. The coach was right.

The Lions' big loss to West Coast was followed by a bye. The club held a meeting at the Gabba where Leigh Matthews spoke to the entire group, and particularly to the wives and girlfriends. He spoke for the first time of winning the premiership in 2003. Until then it had been business as usual. Now it was about history. So he asked the girls for a special effort. He asked them to appreciate the extraordinary situation we were in — one that may never be repeated — and to understand that for the next three months, he hoped, it was going to be full-on football. To accept that maybe at times their partners would neglect them, and overlook home duties and responsibilities.

There wasn't the same immediate on-field improvement that had followed the 2001 and 2002 wake-up calls. We lost three of the next five, to Fremantle, Essendon and Port Adelaide — all by less than nine points. Still, I felt that things were starting to fall into place as August rolled around. We'd had our first bad run of injuries in three years: Jonathan Brown, Clark Keating, Nigel Lappin, Justin

Leppitsch, Tim Notting, Chris Johnson and Beau McDonald had all missed big chunks of football, but we were starting to pull things together.

In Round 19, against Collingwood at the MCG, we wore a Fitzroy-style jumper from the period 1956–73, with the dark blue shoulders and an FFC (Fitzroy Football Club) monogram. Just like Kevin Murray used to wear. It was part of the AFL's Heritage Round, and a timely reminder of where football had come from. It was great for the loyal Fitzroy fans — and great for me, too. The post-game reception at the Hilton was packed, and I'm still astonished that Josie Kelsey, a very loyal supporter, paid the club $12,100 for my signed jumper. The passion in football never ceases to amaze me.

A Round 22 win over the Bulldogs by 86 points consolidated third spot on the ladder, but still we were going to have to do it the hard way. We'd finished second in both 2001 and 2002 and begun our finals campaign at the Gabba. Now we were going to have to start with second-placed Collingwood at the MCG. We lost by 15 points and, worse still, I thought we'd lost Michael Voss for the rest of the year. The captain did his knee in the first quarter and left the stadium on crutches. It would be a miracle if he played again in 2003, I thought.

The loss to Collingwood meant that for the first time in three years we couldn't have the luxury of a week off in the finals. It would be Adelaide at the Gabba in a knockout semi-final just six days later. We beat the Crows by seven goals and were off to Telstra Stadium for a preliminary final date with the Sydney Swans. Another first. In 2001 and 2002 we'd played the grand final qualifier at the Gabba, and after a break. Not this time. When Sydney kicked the last four goals of the third quarter to pull within three points of us, the pundits were writing us off. The end of an era, they said. They're gone.

Momentum was certainly with the Swans, but we'd always prided ourselves on seeing every game right out, and that was the message from the coach at three-quarter time: stick to the plan, do the team things, keep running, keep pushing.

The crowd was unbelievable. More than 70,000 at the home of the Sydney Olympics, where three years earlier Cathy Freeman had stopped the nation to win a gold medal, and all but a handful were wildly chanting Syd-ney, Syd-ney. It's one of those occasions you remember.

Martin Pike played a great final quarter and we kicked 6.6 to 0.1 to win by 44 points. Sydney's Daryn Cresswell retired and was carried from the ground by his teammates.

It was a sad finish for my old mate from Tasmania, but we had other things to worry about.

Midway through the final quarter, Nigel Lappin, running with the flight of the ball, took a heavy knock to the ribs from teammate Shaun Hart. The official post-match medical report told the media he had a corked thigh, but the players knew otherwise. Especially when he was taken to hospital virtually straight after the final siren. I was chosen to replace him for the random drug test.

Filling that little bottle wasn't my only concern. In the second quarter I'd felt my thigh tighten right up, and in the third quarter I felt a twinge. To suggest I feared the worst would be an exaggeration, but I knew it would be another grand final week locked in the medical room as I made sure my thigh was all right.

It was another different grand final build-up. For the second year in a row we would play Collingwood for the flag, but this time they were hot favourites, and fair enough. They'd beaten us in the first final, were coming off a 44-point preliminary final win over minor premiers Port Adelaide, and we had all sorts of injury concerns. 'Happy' Lappin, who finally had something to be sad about, was unlikely to play and Vossy was still carrying his crook knee.

I'd watched the Collingwood–Port game on the afternoon before our game, and one telling thing had happened: Anthony Rocca was reported. His suspension was costly. Nathan Buckley and Chris Tarrant were superstars, but Rocca was the most important player in the Magpie side. He was a big forward who could take a big mark and kick a long goal. And he could give Josh Fraser a spell in the ruck and still be a dangerous target drifting forward.

We tried to keep our grand final week preparation as normal as possible. Why change a winning formula? Except that the medical staff worked double overtime. Nigel Lappin could hardly walk with his broken ribs, but at least there was some hope after a secret test in which a specialist had administered an inter-costal block, effectively numbing the nerve and easing the pain. Vossy didn't do much on his knee, as usual, and I seemed to spend half the week in the hyperbaric chamber trying to get my thigh right. Unknown to most, Jonathan Brown played the entire finals series with a broken hand, and there were others with the customary late-season niggling injuries.

Privately, as I watched *The Footy Show* on television in Melbourne on the Thursday night, I had some doubts.

I didn't quite know what to make of our chances. And although you try not to listen, most in the media were saying the Pies would win. We'd played every week of the finals and travelled three times. Collingwood had had a week off and hadn't left the MCG. And they would have learned from the heartbreaking loss of 2002. I knew we were sore. We were taking injured players into the grand final.

And then I did something I'd never done before: I pulled out a pen and some paper and went through the match-ups. I paired the teams up man for man and turned off the television, convinced I was wrong even to have doubts. Suddenly I felt a lot more confident.

And when Nigel got through a Friday night fitness test after another painkilling session, even surviving some solid tackling from emergency selection Aaron Shattock, I was even more confident. The coach conducted the team meeting on the assumption that Nigel was playing, although we knew the medical staff would have one last look on grand final morning. Chris Scott, the standby player, went to bed not really knowing whether or not he'd be playing.

So off we went to the MCG on a cool but fine day, with only an occasional shower to dampen the turf.

Nothing likely to cause any serious trouble. I was to receive an injection in the top of my thigh to take the spasm out of the muscle. I went for a jog in the rooms to make sure everything was OK and it turned out they hadn't quite got the right spot, so I went looking for Dr Paul McConnell. Bad move. I walked into the coach's room, and there in deep conversation were Leigh, Nigel, physiotherapist Peter Stanton and the doctor. I quickly back-pedalled out the door, and only learned later that just as the coach was about to rule him out, Nigel said he thought he could play. That was good enough for Leigh. He left. Didn't want to give the All-Australian midfielder any time to change his mind.

After all the uncertainty, the team was as selected. Chris Scott, denied a spot in the team in his own right by a bad case of osteitis pubis but dressed, strapped and ready to play if Nigel didn't come up, slowly took off his match gear and joined the brains trust in the coach's box. I can't begin to understand what that would be like. One of those moments when words don't adequately describe the split emotions of team sport.

There were six changes from the 2002 premiership side: Jamie Charman, Ash McGrath and three-game veteran Richard Hadley were in for their first grand final, Robbie

Copeland and Daniel Bradshaw were back for their second after missing selection in 2002, and Blake Caracella was looking forward to his third grand final — his first with the Lions. Missing from 2002 were Chris Scott, twin brother Brad, who had broken his leg in Round 22, Beau McDonald, sidelined since Round 14 by knee problems, plus Tim Notting and Aaron Shattock, who had not been selected, and Des Headland, who had gone to Fremantle.

After two weeks of starting on the bench, Vossy took back his customary spot in the middle. Not that Browny would remember it. He was KO'd by Scott Burns at the first bounce after he'd tapped the ball over his shoulder. From a downfield free kick Simon Black went long and, inside the first minute, I'd marked on my chest and kicked the first goal. It was just the start we needed. And happily, Browny dragged himself to his feet and battled on.

The absence of Rocca from the Collingwood side had forced coach Mick Malthouse to reassess his structure. And that suited me down to the ground. In the qualifying final three weeks earlier, I'd found it difficult to find any space because Jason Cloke was stationed in front of me as a loose man. It wasn't the first time they'd employed these tactics to good effect. Sometimes, even, there were two extra backmen, with Rhyce Shaw being used in a roaming role, and it certainly clogged up our forward set-up — we only kicked one goal after half-time. I was expecting more of the same, but with Rocca missing, Malthouse started Cloke at centre half forward.

It was one of those days where pretty much everything turned to gold for the Lions, and the opposite for the Magpies. We led by 14 points at the first change, and kicked 6.2 to 1.4 in the second term to take a 42-point lead at half-time. By three-quarter time the lead had been cut to 33 points, but it blew out as far as 69 midway through the last quarter.

A telling moment came late in the second term as we capitalised on a few Collingwood errors. I've seen it on television countless times: a long snap over my shoulder for a goal after Rhyce Shaw had fumbled. He was widely castigated in the media for his error, but he was making the right play. A nimble running player should always be able to get around a big fella like me, and that's exactly what he tried to do. The only thing he did wrong was drop the ball. He was unlucky — I could have put it straight out of bounds.

The last 15 minutes, when we knew the game was over, were special. It's a rare treat to know you've got the ultimate prize locked up so early. And for the third year in a row. Craig McRae ran past me and said: 'How good is Mad Monday going to be?' Always thinking, 'Fly'. The official Mad Monday convenor and director of activities, he was probably planning a few games at the same time. We won by 50 points. Jason Akermanis had kicked five goals but Simon Black was a unanimous choice for the Norm Smith Medal, with 39 possessions. Not a bad afternoon's work.

I felt for Rocca. And for Cloke, who had missed the 2002 grand final through suspension. It's a monumental price to pay and neither incident was really nasty. Having faced a similar prospect in 2001, I can just begin to understand what they went through.

In the rooms, I was ready. I pulled out my 2001 and 2002 premiership medallions, which just happened to be in my bag. It was the perfect photograph opportunity, but I can't claim it was any great plan. The fact was, the medals had been sitting on top of the microwave in the kitchen at home from the day I'd won them and as I was about to go out the door, leaving an empty house, I thought, that's not a very safe place to leave them. So I took them with me.

If the overriding post-siren emotion was excitement in 2001 and relief in 2002, in 2003 it was disbelief. We'd won three premierships in a row. This was bigger and better than dreams, because you never imagine you could win three straight. Not since Melbourne in 1955, 1956 and 1957 had any club completed a hat-trick.

All night, as we went through the now familiar celebration routine, the players kept shaking their heads as if they didn't really believe it. I didn't. Yet again, it didn't sink in for me until I took my customary holiday at Mooloolaba a couple of weeks later. Another chance to catch up with the anonymous few who were becoming October regulars. But this year, as well as enjoying the satisfaction of victory, I had a serious question to ponder. I'd been the oldest player in the League in 2003, having turned 35 in June. The fourth-oldest premiership player in history, they'd told me. Retirement was something I needed to think about.

12

MY LAST YEAR

Sitting on the balcony of our unit at Mooloolaba, looking out over the Pacific Ocean during the picture-perfect month of October 2003, I was content with my decision to retire from AFL football. I'd been incredibly fortunate to be part of a club in such an era; I couldn't have asked for more. Three premierships in a row was more than I'd ever dreamed of. I was happy to begin the next phase of my life.

I'd made the decision to give football away just before my family's annual holiday on the Sunshine Coast. I was now out of contract, for the first time in 10 years, and I'd received an offer for 2004 which I felt indicated that I wasn't really wanted. It seemed the club was ready to move on and build for the future. That was understandable.

But deep down, I felt I could play again. After all, I was coming off what had been perhaps my best season of League football. Certainly my best as a stay-at-home full forward. I'd kicked a career-best 78 goals in the Lions' 2003 premiership campaign and finished eighth in the club championship — my best effort in five years under Leigh Matthews. And my health was pretty good. I felt my form and fitness warranted another year, and I wanted to play. I even felt there was room for improvement in my preparation and consistency. And the opportunity to have a crack at winning four flags in a row was never going to come around again.

The initial Brisbane offer for 2004 was about half what I was paid in 2003. But let me be very strong on this point: my decision was never about money. Sure, I wanted to be paid a reasonable sum for the job I was doing. But the important thing for me was whether or not the club really wanted me to play, still considered me a front-line AFL player and a key member of the team.

It seemed to me that their offer was saying that they didn't. I felt they thought I was more a form of insurance — a safety net, perhaps, if things didn't work out. Plan B.

I certainly didn't want to finish my career as a fill-in player, splitting my time between the reserves and the seniors. And no matter how strongly I felt that I was still more valuable than that, I couldn't argue with the club's right to make that decision.

One thing I'd learned was that when your time is up, your time is up. There's very little middle ground. For someone who'd been convinced he was finished in 1995, when CFS took hold, I'd already had eight bonus years. And three premierships. So I told the club I had officially retired and went to the coast to begin thinking about life after football.

One morning not long into my holiday, Leigh Matthews and Graeme Allan came to visit me. Gubby had rung the day before to make sure I was going to be around. We had a coffee. We didn't talk money; we talked football. And over a couple of skinny cappuccinos, the two men who had played such important roles in turning the Brisbane Lions around turned my career around one last time. They convinced me that they really did see a key role for me in 2004, that things wouldn't be any different from the previous years, and that they regarded me as the first-choice full forward.

The sticking point was the salary cap. The Lions were having problems fitting everyone in, and they'd already come up with a means via which I could be paid $100,000 outside the cap — as a Testimonial Year payment. It was totally legal and within AFL guidelines. It fell under a scheme that allows clubs to recognise long-serving players. I wasn't going to get that money until I retired, but that wasn't an issue. The issue was that I didn't want a Testimonial Year.

I wasn't comfortable with the principle of that sort of thing, which is built around the club virtually asking supporters and sponsors to put their hands in their pockets to help pump up a Testimonial Fund. I felt I'd been more than adequately paid for my 10 years in Brisbane, and in a team game I didn't want such a strong individual focus. To have a string of functions that were all about me just didn't sit well. I couldn't do it.

So we reached a compromise. I had a Testimonial Year without any testimonial functions. I accepted the terms the club was offering and they accepted that they wouldn't be able to offset the money via any functions. I finished my holiday and was back in Brisbane for the start of summer training in mid-November.

Marcus Ashcroft, a triple premiership teammate who was three years younger than me, had retired. He didn't have a choice. He was heading for a hip replacement and couldn't possibly have played again. That helped me realise how lucky I was. With an otherwise full playing complement, I knew we were going to be right in the mix again.

At the first team meeting of the summer Leigh produced a picture frame with three photos in it. One of each of the three premiership teams. There was a blank space in the bottom right corner. Written across the top of the frame the coach had put the words, 'I want to be part of four.' And across the bottom it said, 'Do you want to be part of four?'

Summer training was stock-standard for me. Not a lot of time on the track but plenty of work in the pool, in the gym and on the bike. There's no doubt that the year off in 1995 and my inability to do the hard slog that other players went through, pounding the track each summer, had prolonged my career. My joints felt pretty good and I was as fresh as any League footballer of 35 could be.

I felt so good, in fact, that I wasn't prepared to say definitely that 2004 would be my last year. I went into my 17th AFL season with an open mind. As I'd done every year for the last few years, I'd make that decision in October.

But I reckon I set a mark that will probably never be equalled. I completed an entire career's worth of pre-season campaigns, such as they were for the last decade, without doing a beep test. That's the gut-busting endurance test in which you run between two lines 20m apart.

It's a real favourite of the fitness coaches and is done to a recorded beep, starting slowly and getting progressively quicker. You have to turn before the beep each time — if you miss two in a row you're out. The beep test wasn't in vogue in my younger days, and since 1995 I hadn't contemplated it. Not a chance. All I knew about it was that ex-rookie list player Joel Macdonald was throwing down a challenge to the long-time benchmark pair of Shaun Hart and Simon Black.

I hadn't done a 3km time-trial since 1999, when I got over-excited and overdid things in the first summer under Leigh Matthews. I had my routine and the coaching staff were making sure I stuck to it. I made sure I was healthy and let my fitness come through playing games.

But one session in mid-March, a couple of weeks before the start of the premiership, caused a setback that would have ramifications for the entire year. Doing extra work with some young guys and others who hadn't done a lot of training, I tore my thigh muscle. It cost me weeks and, more than that, it cost me a decent fitness base. It left me vulnerable to further soft-tissue injuries as the year wore on and sentenced me to a lot of time in the physio's room. Even more than normal.

There wasn't much the Lions medical staff couldn't beat, but I proved a real challenge for them in 2004. It was to be one injury after another. A thigh, a groin, an ankle, a hamstring and ultimately another thigh. It just goes to show how important a good fitness base is.

I didn't go to Perth in Round 4, but played the next two weeks and then did my ankle against the Kangaroos at Telstra Dome in Round 7. It was one of those odd things. I just landed awkwardly in a marking contest and strained the syndesmosis, one of the ligaments that hold the tibia and fibula together. With the ligament out of commission, the two bones would flare out sideways, so I couldn't put any weight on the ankle. I had four weeks on crutches with a boot-like brace on my ankle, and missed eight weeks. I was underdone before the injury, and I was even more so after it.

Eight weeks on the sidelines mid-season is a long time. Except for when I missed the 1995 campaign, I'd never spent such an infuriatingly long time out of the game. You feel lost. You're part of the club but you're not part of the team. And no matter how hard they try to include you in what's going on, the reality is that you're just making up the numbers.

If there was a time when I knew 2004 would be my last season it was during this period. There was no definitive moment. It just happened. I was realistic enough to admit that I wasn't doing enough to warrant another year: this was it.

I returned in Round 14, and then in the third quarter of the Round 18 against Sydney at the SCG, I strained my groin. Two more weeks out of action. I'd played nine of the first 20 games and hadn't finished two of them.

Round 16, against Collingwood at the MCG, was my 300th. To be honest, it wasn't a big thing for me. In the years ahead I'm sure I'll be proud to have reached such a major milestone, particularly as two of my best mates, Paul Roos and John Blakey, had already done so. But it certainly wasn't a factor in my decision to play on in 2004.

The best part of my 300th game was taking Madison and Tom through the banner. Claudia, who was a week short of her first birthday, stayed at home with my mum, but the older kids, six and four by now, had a great time, decked out in their No. 11 Lions jumpers. A few of their mates saw them on television so they were pretty happy. Watching the people in the grandstand while enjoying chips and drinks was a bit of a treat, too. More often than not, for them, football at the Gabba meant an afternoon in the crèche with the other players' kids or a night at home with the babysitter. We didn't take them out to night games because they would usually be asleep by the time the game started.

No sooner had Pete taken the kids off the ground than it started to hail. A special storm for the start of my 300th game. Looking back towards the city I could see the sheets of hail coming in over the top of the grandstand. It was a serious storm and all I got was cold — I didn't see a lot of the ball in the first quarter. The storm stopped at the break but it wasn't a great night for marking forwards. I finished with three goals in a handy six-goal win.

I did appreciate a few of the little things on the night. For instance, after I'd spent time on the bench with cramp in the last quarter, Leigh Matthews put me back for the last few seconds so I could finish on the ground. And teammate Martin Pike grabbed the match ball immediately after the final siren and stuffed it up his jumper to hide it from the umpires. You can always rely on Martin to be on the ball. He must have remembered what had happened in the 2001 grand final. I appreciated, too, the fact that Leigh waited on the boundary line to shake my hand after the game. And that he presented the match ball to me in the rooms afterwards. They are the things that make milestone games special.

We always made a point after the game of going to where the bulk of the Lions supporters were sitting to acknowledge them, and that allowed me to pay tribute to the people who had stuck by me for so long. I even spotted my No. 1 fans, the old Lynch Mob, before Michael Voss and Justin Leppitsch somehow carried me 100m to the boundary line.

Back at the team hotel I caught up with family and friends. This time my two brothers were there, and that didn't happen often. At my wedding, Vaughan was at sea with his job in the merchant navy, and at Vaughan's wedding, Manuel, who served as an electrical weapons technician in the Australian Navy, was on HMAS *Brisbane* in the Gulf War.

Though I had a frustrating year with injury, the team was pretty consistent. Only once did we drop outside the top three on the ladder, after Round 6. The annual wake-up call had come in Round 9, against Fremantle in Perth — they thumped us by 59 points. It was the first time since the 2003 wake-up call that the opposition had kicked 20 goals, and it served to once more remind everyone of the formula that had proved so successful: play your role, don't try to be or do anything more, worry about the process and the results will look after themselves.

I returned from injury (again) in Round 21, when a Gabba win over St Kilda locked up a top two spot for us. The Saints had been unbeaten through the first 10 rounds after winning the Wizard Cup and were premiership favourites for much of the year, so to beat them by 45 points in the run to the finals was a positive sign.

So was a 113-point win over the Kangaroos in Round 22, but for me the game was a disaster. I was doing fine — I had four goals — until I made a full-pace lead 21 minutes into the third term. I dived forward to take the chest mark, and in the last stride I did my hamstring. I knew it had gone so I walked straight off the ground. It was a disappointing way for me to finish my 98th — and last, as it turned out — game at the Gabba. There was no opportunity for a final farewell, so to the multitudes of Brisbane fans who treated me so well over the years, thank you so much. You were very kind to me. Even when I was sick or wasn't going well the fans were sensational, and their support really did make a difference.

The diagnosis was: no chance the first week of the finals, some hope for the second and probable for the third. And, as history would show, they were spot on.

I watched from the stands as the Lions belted St Kilda by 80 points in the qualifying final at the Gabba. It was a sensational performance and a huge confidence booster. I started to think we really were on track for a fourth flag. The football pundits around the country were probably saying the same thing. Here they come. The triple premiers are just tuning up for September. And that's exactly how it felt.

The week off was good for me. It made sure my hamstring was right. I'd had a good week on the track and went into the preliminary final against Geelong at the MCG in pretty good shape. I was seeing the ball well and took a few good marks, but I also missed some simple chances. Luckily, it didn't cost us. We hung on to beat a really good young Geelong side by nine points.

The win came at a price: Shaun Hart had suffered cheekbone and jaw fractures in a horrific third-quarter collision with teammate Daniel Bradshaw when he was running with the flight of the ball. It was typical of the courage of Harty, one of the smallest players in the game. It turned out to be a very sad end to a magnificent 273-game career.

I borrowed Leigh Matthews' car on the Sunday morning and took Justin Leppitsch and Simon Black with me to visit Harty in Epworth Hospital. He didn't look as bad as I thought he might have looked, but his face was very swollen. He wasn't able to fly for a few days so the club flew his wife and two sons to Melbourne and they spent grand final week in a serviced apartment in Kew.

The win had been another historic moment for the Lions: our first preliminary final win in Melbourne. We were through to our fourth consecutive grand final. Brisbane against Port Adelaide. The first grand final without a Victoria-based side.

Whether or not we should have had to play the preliminary final at the MCG was part of an ongoing debate. For the first time a non-Victorian club had lost the hard-earned right to host the grand final qualifier because of the 42-year agreement between the AFL and the MCC to play at least one preliminary final each year at the MCG.

Notwithstanding that, we had a good — albeit short — preparation. Jonathan Brown carried a knee problem and Craig McRae a hamstring worry that would see them having Friday morning fitness tests, but otherwise we were in good shape. Even the old fella who played at full forward. It was ironic that after three grand finals in which I'd really struggled to get on the paddock, I was better going into the 2004 decider following a nightmare season with injury.

I walked from the team base at the Parkview Hotel up St Kilda Road to Wesley College for the fitness tests for Browny and Fly. I didn't want to be cooped up in my room all day doing nothing and I wanted to show the boys some support. Oddly, it took me back to my teenage days. There was a junior soccer clinic on, so while the boys warmed up I kicked a soccer ball around with some kids. I always thought Browny would play — it was just a question of how long he would last and how effective he would be. But I got a pleasant surprise when Fly came up. Another win for the physios and co.

So we went in with four changes from the 2003 grand final. Jamie Charman, injured in Round 17, was a big loss. Likewise Harty, who had joined us for dinner at the team hotel on the Thursday night. Marcus Ashcroft had retired and Ash McGrath wasn't selected. In their place were the 2001–02 premiership trio of Brad Scott, Chris Scott and Tim Notting, plus grand final rookie Dylan McLaren.

The bookies found it hard to work out who was going to win. Would the experience of the Lions outweigh the impact of the injury worries and tough preparation and see us through to a fourth consecutive flag? Or would Port, in their first AFL grand final after three years in a row on top of the ladder, finally break through?

Players try to prepare for everything in a grand final, but there are things you just can't anticipate. Like a torn quad muscle 15 minutes in.

I led to the pocket in front of the Great Southern Stand at the city end of the MCG. In the last two strides my thigh went. It didn't matter that Port captain Warren Tredrea, pushing back from his position at the opposite end, had taken the mark. For me the damage was done. I was devastated. This was meant to be the biggest game of my life, and instead it turned out to be the most disappointing. This was not the way it was meant to end.

I can't explain what happened in the next minute or so. I'd signalled to the bench that I was gone and I found myself out of the play. There was the customary niggling from my opponent Darryl Wakelin that is always frustrating. It's something you put up with 99 per cent of the time, but this time I just lashed out at him. The frustration of knowing that my last game was effectively over before it had begun got the better of me. I guess it says something about the emotion of grand final day.

I was only pleased that I didn't do any damage. Perhaps it was my subconscious working. I'd like to think so, because it's not the way I played my football for 17 years, and not the way it should be played. It was embarrassing.

It certainly wasn't a conscious action and I deeply regret it, but I have to take responsibility for my actions.

I spent the rest of the grand final trying to defy inevitability. The medical staff tried a couple of local anaesthetic injections to settle down my quad but it was no good. I could jog all right but when I returned to the ground in the second and third quarters I couldn't get above half pace. When Leigh Matthews asked me at the final change if there was any hope I had to shake my head. I was no good.

So I spent the last quarter of my last match on the bench, praying that somehow we could overcome a 17-point three-quarter time deficit. It had been a close struggle. Port kicked the first three goals, but in the second quarter we got four quick ones to get seven points up. We led by a point at half-time and by six points 10 minutes later. The Power, though, got the next four goals and finished with nine of the last 10. Our blokes were out on their feet.

As soon as the siren sounded I made my way to Darryl Wakelin in the middle of the ecstatic Port huddle. I congratulated him on his game and his side's win, and he was good enough to offer his congratulations on my career. Then I left him to his celebrations. We'd had some mighty battles over the years but there was no doubting the winner this time. All credit to him, and to Port coach Mark

Williams and his entire team. They were too quick and too good on the day, and were deserving premiers. In that group I include injured captain Matthew Primus and Josh Francou. To win despite missing two All-Australian players for virtually the entire year made it an even better effort.

Watching the presentations is tough, but you have to do it. Essendon in 2001 and Collingwood in 2002–03 had done the same thing while we enjoyed our moment of glory. Walking off the MCG it hit me that I'd never be back as a player.

Inside, Leigh Matthews spoke to the players one last time in the coach's room. I've got no idea what he said because I had something else on my mind. I hadn't planned to announce my retirement, but it just struck me as we walked into the room that this may be the last time the entire group was together in an appropriate environment. The time was right. It had to be now.

So as soon as Leigh finished I said, 'I've just got something to say.' As I stood up in front of the group I wondered exactly what it was going to be. I don't think it was any surprise, because everyone pretty much knew it would be my last game — and if they didn't, Jason Akermanis had told everyone during the week in his newspaper column. But that didn't make it any easier to get the words out.

I really struggled to speak at first. Even through the tears welling in my eyes I could see tears all around the room, and that didn't make it any easier. But once I got started I battled through. I told the players how, after 17 years, the time was right to give it away. This was the moment when it really sank in. I told them how much it meant to me to have played with such an incredible team, and such an incredible group of people. That's why it was so sad. These guys weren't just teammates; it went much, much deeper than that. They were people I'd spent countless hours with over many years, working together for a common goal. People with whom I'd shared three extraordinary premierships. People for whom everyone in the room would have done anything. They were people I respected greatly. And people I knew I was going to really miss. Nobody said a word. At least I don't think they did.

But the job wasn't done yet. I still had to face the media. It wasn't pleasant, but I had to tell them, and through them the football public, that I'd given it away. I did my best to answer the questions of the newspaper reporters first and then did a couple of radio interviews. It's much easier when you've won.

In the dressing rooms, hardly anyone had moved. Most sat there, still in their match gear, staring blankly into space. And those who had changed were sitting in front of their locker doing the same thing. What a contrast it was to the three previous years.

Afterwards I caught up with Peta, family and friends. Mum and her partner Peter had come down from the Sunshine Coast, Dad was up from Queenstown, Manuel had come from Devonport, and Vaughan was down from Bundaberg. Plus Pete's father Neil. At least there was one good thing — I wouldn't have to try to find so many grand final tickets ever again. That had always been a struggle, and we only managed to get everyone along this time because Mum, who had been a Gabba regular, borrowed membership tickets from a few friends who were not intending to go and joined the long queue to buy grand final tickets outside the Gabba on the Sunday morning after the preliminary final.

The grand final dinner at the Crown Casino was, predictably, a flat affair. I was feeling as crook as I had for a long time. I think it was a reaction to the local anaesthetics I'd been given during the game. Whatever, I wasn't well enough to drink, had hardly anything to eat, and had to decline an invitation to do an interview with Master of Ceremonies Craig Willis. I felt bad about that, but I just couldn't have done it.

Learning from the lessons of years past, when getting a taxi at the casino after the dinner was next to mission impossible, we'd booked a limo to pick us up at 2am. By then, Peta and I were more than happy to sneak off. Appropriately enough, we gave Peter Stanton a ride back to the hotel. The physiotherapist who had looked after me so diligently and so magnificently for six years was just finishing off the job.

On Sunday morning the numbers were down a bit at Brunswick Street, but still pretty good. And the spirit among the fans was fantastic. One group of supporters even managed to put a smile on my face. The Lynch Mob was there in force, and they presented me with the banner which they'd waved in the outer all those years. It was a terrific gesture, and I look forward to the time when I can get to the football and buy them a few beers — which I undoubtedly owe them. Then it was back to the Gabba for one last farewell.

Wednesday was the official debriefing. The last time our group would be together. It brought another surprise: Shaun Hart's retirement. A couple of months earlier Harty had told me privately that he was almost certain he'd give it away at the end of the season, but after the horrific accident in the preliminary final he'd changed his mind.

He'd been to see the coach and told him he wanted to play on. However, Leigh had explained that salary cap pressures wouldn't allow it. Shaun accepted the decision in the team-first manner which typified his entire career, and said his thank you and goodbye in style.

I'd made a feeble attempt to clean out my locker, which was full of junk from I don't know when. I took the important stuff, but it was a few weeks before I picked up a box containing the rest of it — my old Tassie mate Shane Johnson had saved it for me.

On the Thursday night I had an appointment with the AFL Tribunal, having been charged two days earlier on video evidence. It was done via video link between Brisbane and Melbourne. I pleaded guilty to attempting to strike Darryl Wakelin but not to striking, because as anyone who had seen the incident would testify, it was largely a lot of air swings. I told the tribunal that Wakelin should not have been made to account for his actions: he was only defending himself. He was fined $5000 for attempting to strike me. I was found guilty on two counts of striking and four counts of attempted striking and was suspended for four matches and three matches on the striking offences, and for three matches for one attempted strike. I was fined $5000 each for the other three attempted strikes. In total, a few nonsensical seconds had cost me $15,000 in fines and a 10-match suspension — which was meaningless unless I was contemplating a comeback, which I wasn't.

I fully expected a decent whack, because I'd done the wrong thing, but I thought the penalty was a bit stiff. After all, there was no damage done. If I'd still been playing I would have appealed the severity of the penalty. After I'd taken one last opportunity to apologise for my actions via the media crew waiting outside I was happy to put the entire incident behind me. Cop it and move on.

There was one more official duty to attend to: the club championship dinner on Saturday night at the Brisbane Convention Centre. This involved 1200 people. I knew I was going to have to make one last speech, and wasn't too confident I'd get through it. Sitting with fellow retiree Craig McRae, I was filthy when he told me early in the night that he'd actually pre-recorded his speech during the week. Why didn't I think of that? When it got to the farewell part of the evening, Harty, dressed for the occasion in a black afro wig, sunglasses and a green suit, went first. Then came Fly, who was wearing black leather pants which must have been painted on, with a fake moustache and a long hairpiece. He didn't say too much — just signalled to run the tape. Then it was my turn. The club had put together a video tribute to music for each of us, but I made sure I didn't look at it as I walked up to the stage. I got through all right, hoping desperately that I wouldn't miss anyone important. It was actually good to have a chance to thank a lot of people and bring to a formal end my 17 years in the AFL. It had been an extraordinary ride. At least now I wasn't the oldest player in the competition. In 2005 that distinction would belong to St Kilda's Robert Harvey.

I had a few beers, but not too many — I wanted to enjoy the occasion, just as I had on our three winning grand final nights. I was rapt that Nigel Lappin won the Merrett/Murray Medal. He'd been around the mark so many times, only to be denied a real chance by injury or narrowly beaten by superstars like Michael Voss, Simon Black, Jason Akermanis and Justin Leppitsch. Nigel deserved to win one. He's his own harshest critic is 'Happy', but it even brought a smile to his face.

About 2am in typical form Peta and I snuck off. We had another engagement. Long past the days of going to 21st birthdays, we did what old football couples do — we went to the 40th birthday party of our regular babysitter, Tizi. I fell into bed about 4.30am, content that the professional football phase of my life was over. I slept well.

13

IT'S ABOUT THE PEOPLE

When I started out, heading to Melbourne in the hope of playing in the AFL for Fitzroy, I had no idea of what the next 17 years would present — especially of the ups and downs, or the sharp learning curve of life. Often our success is measured in wins and losses, assets and other tangible possessions. But the thing that has meant most to me is the people I've met and the experiences I've shared with them.

I was terribly fortunate to enjoy a lot of success in the latter years of my career with the Brisbane Lions, and I will share a life-time bond with the people I was involved with on and off the field. But that is matched by the same friendships from my days with the Fitzroy Lions in

Melbourne. They are friendships that have remained with me despite the fact that we have been spread all over the country.

So, as I do what I always said I'd never do — reflect in a forum such as this on 17 years in the AFL — I count my blessings that I'm joyously wealthy in terms of family, friends and personal experiences.

When I think of moments that others might classify as individual highlights, I recall not the individual satisfaction but the shared enjoyment that comes with being part of a successful team. I know precisely why former world tennis No. 1 Pat Rafter enjoyed playing Davis Cup for Australia so much — because when he was successful he had teammates to share it with. I can imagine that success in an individual sport, as rewarding as it undoubtedly is considering the mountain of hard work that has gone into it, might just be a little hollow. Because outside your immediate family and support network, you don't really have anyone to share it with. Certainly not the same way you do as a member of a successful team.

During my career I was involved in two other great teams. The Fitzroy Team of the Century dinner on Thursday, 3 May 2001, was a night I'll never forget. To see so many people so passionate about the Fitzroy Football Club together for one last time was incredible. It was a magnificent occasion, not because I was chosen among this illustrious group but because I got to share the moment with people who are true legends of the game.

The celebration meant different things to different people. For the many who had embraced the Brisbane–Fitzroy merger it was a huge party; for those who hadn't, it was proof that the 'new' Lions really were genuine about ensuring that Fitzroy lived on, and that the Fitzroy history and tradition really were still alive. And for those who were somewhere in the middle of the emotional tug-of-war, it was a kind of closure — either an official end to Fitzroy or a new beginning with the Brisbane Lions. For me, it was the final glue which brought the two clubs together, never to be separated.

The night covered every different emotion imaginable. More than 1200 people packed the Grand Hyatt Hotel in Melbourne for not one function, but two. The main dinner for 800 was sold out so quickly the club booked the adjacent 400-seat room for people who had been unable to get a seat in the major function room, but were content to watch the presentation live on a big screen from next door. Plus, there was a waiting list of another 200.

The Lions were playing Geelong at the Gabba on the Saturday night. Ordinarily, the last thing I'd do is make an extra flight interstate, but this was special. I was given permission by Leigh Matthews to go to Melbourne. I didn't know in advance that I'd been selected in the side, but the fact that the club had gone to considerable lengths to get me there raised my hopes a little. Peta travelled to Melbourne with me, and when we got to our table we had a pleasant surprise — Dad, who runs the Mount Lyell Motor Inn in Queenstown, had flown up from Tasmania for the night. I started to think that I might be a chance, although he insisted that he knew nothing.

A few years earlier I'd been chosen in the Fitzroy Team of the Half-Century and I'd figured I might be somewhere in the mix, but this time they were choosing 24 players from the 1156 who had represented the club through 1928 AFL matches and eight premierships between 1897 and 1996. It was really special to hear my name called out for this one.

All 16 living members of the team — headed by 79-year-old Brownlow medallist Allan Ruthven, 74-year-old Norm Johnstone and 73-year-old Bill Stephen — were there. At 32, I was the youngest; this was a nice change for me in the latter years of my career. And I was the only one still playing.

I knew all the names, but I hadn't met most of my new teammates. I loved chatting about the good old days as we gathered behind the stage to sign the mass of Team of the Century memorabilia. I was like a kid in a candy store, sharing the moment with four ex-teammates: Paul Roos, Gary Pert, Mick Conlan and Richard Osborne.

I'd heard a lot about Norm Johnstone, a 228-gamer from 1944–57, in particular how tough he was. Yet when he accepted his selection he was crying with pride. It said a lot about how much the night meant to those people.

I can't imagine what sort of job it would have been to select the side, but even I could have picked the captain. Kevin 'Bulldog' Murray, the 1969 Brownlow medallist, was a shoo-in. He won nine Fitzroy best and fairest awards, sharing with South Melbourne's Bob Skilton the record of most wins by any player in any AFL club.

There was barely a dry eye in the place as the old Fitzroy song was sung time and again until late in the evening after the team had been announced and presented.

Each member of the Team of the Century received a beautifully framed listing of the team, complete with a 9-carat gold-plated medallion, plus an autographed and framed copy of the commemorative Team of the Century painting, done by my ex-housemate Jamie Cooper. He had done a corresponding job for most AFL clubs, but this held special significance for the 26-game Fitzroy wingman from 1984–87, so he snuck himself into the painting. He was one of the guys holding up the banner as the players ran through it.

The Fitzroy Team of the Century was:

B: *Bill Stephen, Fred Hughson, Frank Curcio*
HB: *Kevin Murray (c), Paul Roos, Gary Pert*
C: *Warwick Irwin, John Murphy, Wilfred Smallhorn*
HF: *Owen Abrahams, Bernie Quinlan, Garry Wilson (vc)*
F: *Norm Brown, Jack Moriarty, Allan Ruthven*
R: *Alan Gale, Norm Johnstone, Haydn Bunton*
INT: *Mick Conlan, Richard Osborne, Percy Trotter,*
Alastair Lynch, Harvey Merrigan, Percy Parratt
COACH: *Len Smith*

To be chosen in one Team of the Century was incredible; to be chosen in two is still something I cannot quite comprehend. Yet on the night of Friday, 25 June 2004, at Wrest Point Casino in Hobart, it happened when Tasmanian football honoured 25 players, a coach and an umpire.

I have to confess that this time I did know in advance. It was the weekend of the AFL bye, but still there was a lot of work to be done to get everyone there. And when artist extraordinaire Jamie Cooper asked me if I wanted to appear in the Team of the Century painting with the old 'mullet' hairstyle or the more conservative style of latter years, I had a fair idea that I'd been selected.

Still, I had no idea of the huge honour that would come my way with the selection: I was named in a forward pocket next to my old mate and mentor Peter Hudson. Sharing the couch with the great Huddo for an interview with noted Tasmanian football commentator Tim Lane at the dinner was unbelievable.

It was an incredible side. How about the goal-to-goal line — Bob 'Tassie' Johnson, Laurie Nash, Ian Stewart, Royce Hart and Huddo? This time the captaincy would have been a much tougher decision, although you would never argue with their decision: Darrel Baldock. Judging by how he was still holding fort at the bar, a Cascade in his hand, when Peta and I went to bed about 3am, I'd say it was an inspired choice.

This time I wasn't the youngest member of the side — Sydney pair Paul Williams and Daryn Cresswell and Richmond's Matthew Richardson were younger than me.

The Tasmanian Team of the Century was:

B: *Verdun Howell (St K)*, *Bob 'Tassie' Johnson (Melb)*,
Ivor Warne-Smith (Melb)

HB: *Barry Lawrence (St K)*, *Laurie Nash (SM)*,
Brent Crosswell (Carl/NM)

C: *Rodney Eade (Haw)*, *Ian Stewart (St K/Rich)*,
Arthur Hodgson (Carl)

HF: *Darrel Baldock (St K — c)*, *Royce Hart (Rich)*,
Daryn Cresswell (Syd)

F: *Horrie Gorringe (Cananore, Tas)*, *Peter Hudson
(Haw)*, *Alastair Lynch (Fitz/Bris)*

FOLL: *Peter 'Percy' Jones (Carl)*, *John Leedham
(Nth Hobart/Nth Launceston — vc)*, *Terry Cashion
(New Town/Clarence/Longford/Sandy Bay)*

INT: *Paul Williams (Coll/Syd)*, *Len Pye
(Nth Hobart/Fitz/New Norfolk)*, *Matthew Richardson
(Rich)*, *Darrin Pritchard (Haw)*, *Rex Garwood
(New Town/Glenorchy)*, *Michael Roach (Rich)*, *Neil
Conlan (New Town/Devonport)*

COACH: *Roy Cazaly*

A/COACH: *Robert Shaw*

UMPIRE: *Scott Jeffery*

The moment which gave me most pride, though, was in mid-July 2004, when I got a call from my old mate Matty Armstrong in Hobart. He was coach of the Tassie Devils team that played in the VFL — effectively the AFL Reserves competition — and had been sent on a mission by the Tasmanian Football League heavyweights: to seek my permission for a change in football history. They wanted to rename the state's top individual award in my honour.

I'd played in the TFL in 1986–87, when players aspired to win the William Leitch Medal. It had been named after a man regarded as the father of Tasmanian football. He'd begun as a player in 1880 and was later an umpire and administrator until the early 1930s, after being awarded life membership of the Australian Football Council in 1929.

The William Leitch Medal was initially awarded to the best and fairest player in the Hobart-based southern competition, and in the mid–1980s it became the symbol of individual supremacy in the statewide competition.

Among a multitude of winners was Peter Hudson, who won it in 1978 and 1979 after his final fling with Hawthorn in 1977. My first Tasmanian state coach, Andy Bennett, a former Hawthorn and St Kilda player, won it in

1986, and my Bears teammate Adrian Fletcher topped the vote count in 1988 before Scott Wade, now the general manager of Football Tasmania, completed a 1984 and 1989 double. Among the earlier winners were dual Melbourne premiership player and All-Australian Stuart Spencer, who won it in 1960 and 1967, and ex-Hawthorn player and Geelong coach Rod Olsson (1971 and 1973).

When Matty told me, much to my surprise, that they wanted to rename it the Alastair Lynch Medal, I quickly replied, 'What do they want to do that for?' To which Matty said, 'That's what I said to them.' To have something that was such a huge part of Tasmanian football named after me took a lot of comprehending.

I understand the decision was taken to make the medal something which current players could more easily associate with. Though William Leitch was a legend of Tasmanian football, he was from the early days. It just so happened that in the week I was scheduled to become the first Tasmanian to play 300 games the milestone prompted the powers that be to make a change. I didn't have to think twice.

I look forward to presenting the Alastair Lynch Medal every year from now on, but unfortunately I was unable to present the first one to Tassie Devils fullback Matthew

Jovanovic because the dinner coincided with my commitment to the Brisbane Lions 2004 club championship night.

The Lions club championship night was something I could not miss, because it was the final official farewell to a group of people who meant an enormous amount to me. Not just the players, but the whole football club. Fitzroy had meant so much to me for my first six years, and the Brisbane Bears/Lions had meant just as much for the next 11 years.

As I prepared my speech for that last night I was terrified I was going to leave someone out, and it's the same thing now. Everyone plays their part in a successful club, and from the chairman to the boot-studder I'll be forever grateful to them all.

I've tried to mention all who have played official roles but there are many more. They are too numerous to mention by name — they know who they are and are no less appreciated.

I could go on about every one of the 189 different players I played with at club level, plus all the state players, but the 27 players with whom I shared the ultimate football triumph will always be extra special. From the youngest member of the 2001 premiership side,

Jonathan Brown, whom I met when he was a seven-year-old autograph hunter in the Fitzroy dressing rooms in my first season of AFL, to guys like Chris Scott and Nigel Lappin, who had joined the club at the same time I did.

I won't, because there are too many of them. Suffice it to say that the premiership bond with Jason Akermanis, Marcus Ashcroft, Simon Black, Daniel Bradshaw, Jonathan Brown, Blake Caracella, Jamie Charman, Robert Copeland, Richard Hadley, Shaun Hart, Des Headland, Chris Johnson, Clark Keating, Nigel Lappin, Justin Leppitsch, Beau McDonald, Ashley McGrath, Craig McRae, Mal Michael, Tim Notting, Martin Pike, Luke Power, Brad Scott, Chris Scott, Aaron Shattock, Michael Voss and Darryl White is one that will never be broken.

Just as a bunch of former Fitzroy players became special ongoing friends, I suspect the same thing will happen with the Brisbane players. Different ages and different circumstances will take people down different paths. We may not see each other every second week, but there will always be a sense of pride and satisfaction among the entire group, a group which learned the secret of winning from the depths of defeat and despair, and put together an era of modern football the likes of which we may never see again.

*   *   *

But special memories for me are not just those related to success or recognition. And they're not just about football. Not at all. I also remember fondly a whole string of other experiences because of the people they involved.

Brisbane has grown up so much, even in my short time north of the Tweed River, and it offers two things that I cherish — a sporting smorgasbord and a wonderful environment in which to raise children. As much as I loved my first 19 years in Tasmania and my next six years in Melbourne, I'm firmly entrenched now in the Sunshine state. My three children were all born here. They visit friends and family interstate, but to them Brisbane is home.

For Peta and me that's a big change from when we moved to Brisbane in October 1993. At that time I expected to play six or seven years with the Bears, work for the club for three or four years to complete my 10-year contract, and then move back to Melbourne. However, the longer you stay in a place the more settled you become and the harder it is to leave.

Probably the thing that has changed most during my time in Queensland is AFL football. Not long after I'd arrived in Brisbane I did a clinic at a school in South Brisbane. I was introduced to a bunch of kids aged seven and eight on the oval and got a pretty rude awakening. One young kid said to me, 'You're rubbish — where's Alfie?' The person he wanted in my place was Brisbane Broncos captain Allan 'Alfie' Langer. I learned pretty quickly just where AFL football sat in the pecking order in Brisbane.

The move of the Bears from Carrara to Brisbane was one of two things that really turned AFL football around in southeast Queensland. The other was the decision by the then Bears to change their recruiting focus to youth. This was pivotal, and people like Robert Walls, coach at the time, and recruiting managers Scott Clayton and Kinnear Beatson should take a lot of the credit for the success of the club in more recent times.

Brisbane is a unique city in sporting terms because all the sporting teams are part of a common family — they are rivals and allies at the same time. They compete and co-exist, if that's possible. Almost like a fraternity. It's not like in Melbourne, where the 10 AFL sides compete against each other. Where the culture is football, football, football. Where the game will always prosper because it is the main game. In Brisbane there is no AFL rival for the Lions; instead, the opposition is the Broncos, the

Queensland Reds (rugby union), the Queensland Bulls (cricket), the Brisbane Bullets (basketball), the new Queensland Roar (soccer's A-League), and anyone else who plays in a national competition.

The different teams are rivals for the corporate and membership dollar, and for media time and space, but otherwise we get on famously. In the last few years Leigh Matthews organised a three-codes football luncheon for the Lions, Broncos and Reds, where every player from each side attended to raise money for the charity of choice of each club. It was always a good day.

I loved the cross-code interaction. One of a number of special highlights for me was the Carl Rackemann celebrity day/night cricket match in January 1995 at ANZ Stadium, home of the 1982 Brisbane Commonwealth Games. It was part of the testimonial year celebrations for Rackemann and brought together a plethora of international cricketing stars and local sporting identities.

Spending time in the company of cricketing greats such as Greg Chappell, Dennis Lillee, Viv Richards, Gus Logie, Dean Jones, Stuart Law and, of course, Rackemann. There was also a host of people from other sports doing what I was doing — enjoying the occasion and trying not to make too big a goose of myself.

I opened the bowling with the guest of honour himself, which was a lot of fun, but batting was always going to be a different proposition. As I walked out, late in the innings, I was greeted partway to the wicket by the great man himself, Viv Richards. He wasn't my batting partner — he was the bowler. And I was awfully glad it was Viv and his slow little tweakers rather than a pace demon like Malcolm Marshall or Michael Holding. When I got within earshot he said to me, 'Where do you want it?' With 17,000 people watching and my heart rate up around 200 beats per minute, I told him, 'A little nude one outside off-stump would be tremendous, thanks.' And that's exactly where he put it, just so I could get one in the middle and pat it straight back to him. It was a generous gesture.

It was a great experience and something I'll never forget, but it did take its toll. It occurred before I'd had the CFS diagnosis and still didn't know what was wrong with me, and two overs bowling and only a few more with the bat had wiped me out. When the rest of the players caught a bus into town to continue the post-match festivities I headed home to bed. And there I stayed for the best part of the next week. It was disappointing to miss what would have been a lot of fun, but I was exhausted.

Another of my favourite sporting memories is the day in 2002 when I played one hole of golf with Greg Norman. I'd been asked to help Norman launch one of his club-based competitions, at Pelican Waters Golf Course at Caloundra on the Sunshine Coast. The Shark played one hole with each group in the field. I've never been more nervous standing on the tee with a golf club in my hand.

Afterwards, we had a fantastic chat. Greg was a former No. 1 ticket-holder of the Brisbane Bears and knew all about the club and the Lions' 2001 premiership. He asked more questions than he answered, which was tremendous. Even though he lives in the United States, he obviously keeps in close contact with what is happening in Australia.

That's typical of the comradeship and spirit that exist between sportsmen. And it's not just restricted to Australian shores. On the 1999 Lions end-of-season trip I bumped into Queensland and Australian rugby players Tim Horan and Chris Latham in Ireland. It was during the Rugby World Cup, and Australia were scheduled to play Ireland at Lansdowne Road. I remember it well, because outside the gate on game day I came across a lady rattling a collection tin looking to raise money for research into ME, otherwise known as chronic fatigue syndrome!

A couple of days before the World Cup clash, a bunch of keen golfers in the Lions group had booked a game at Portmarnock, one of the top links courses in the world. There were Chris and Brad Scott, my fellow Tasmanian Trent Bartlett, and me. We had a 9am tee-off so we got up early to get across town to the course. Who do we bump into in the carpark but Horan and Latham. I'd met them both through various promotions and we had a good chat before they headed off to the pro shop as we unpacked our gear.

Inside, I asked the guy at the counter where we had to pay. He must have picked the accent because he said immediately, 'Are you with the Australians?' What could I say? 'Yes, we're with the Australians,' I told him, which wasn't totally untrue. 'How many of you are coming?' he asked. With that I said to Tim, who was still in the pro shop 'How many are coming today?' Reading the play beautifully, he said, 'Six, I think.' There were six — him, Chris, the Scott twins, big Bart and me. 'No worries — just go to the clubhouse, sign the visitors' book and you're away,' said the guy behind the counter. It was something like A$200 a round, so we'd done nicely.

Then we had to sign in. Thinking we'd better go with some Wallaby players, I opted for the name Jason Little.

Not a bad choice, because on a dark night we might actually look vaguely similar. Chris Scott signed in as Ben Tune and Brad Scott chose Dan Herbert, but big Bart hesitated. The 193cm pale-skinned Tasmanian didn't know a lot of Wallabies, and we thought his first choice of John Eales wasn't so smart. He was pretty well known. So what did Bart come up with? Toutai Kefu. If you don't know Toutai Kefu, he's a massive man, not dissimilar in stature to Bart, but he's of Tongan extraction. Hardly likely to be confused with the boy from Deloraine in northern Tasmania. As we left the clubhouse we were a little concerned that a bunch of 12- and 13-year-old kids nearby may have been onto us, but we got away unscathed.

We had a great day, and just as we were about to leave, having dropped the buggies back to the pro shop, the guy behind the counter said, 'Hang on, fellas — the captain of the club has just arrived and I'm sure he'd like to say hello.' As it turned out, he had invited the Wallabies to play at Portmarnock. And worse still, he had played for Ireland against Australia and was good mates with a certain Wallabies captain of the mid-1960s.

I can't remember who it was, but I've since learned that John Thornett was Wallabies skipper in 1965, so let's say it was him. One thing I did know for sure was that we were in trouble.

'You'd know John Thornett,' said the club captain. 'Not personally,' I replied, feeling worse by the second, struggling not to choke on my words. 'But I know him by reputation, of course. He was a great player.'

Somehow, we managed to fudge our way through without being totally humiliated, though as we drove away we decided they were probably onto us. Brad Scott had bought a new driver and paid for it with his own credit card.

Next day we played at the Portmarnock Hotel course, which was a newer course, but just as much fun. This time we really were invited guests of the Wallabies, who were staying on the course. And who do you think invited us? Toutai Kefu.

I've also shared many a game of golf with the ex-Fitzroy trio of Paul Roos, Gary Pert and John Blakey. It was always the pretty boys, Roos and Pert, against the battlers, Lynch and Blakey. Johnny and I have won our share, but we don't really have anything much to show for it. Nothing to fire back with when Roosy and Perty come to visit and say, 'Remember that day in Tassie when Johnny hit that one into the carpark . . .!'

Now, it doesn't seem quite as important. Life isn't just about winning and losing, and it's certainly not about trophies and collectables. It's about happy and healthy time spent with friends and family. And believe me, you don't fully appreciate that until it is taken away from you.

14

LIFE AFTER FOOTBALL

Professional footballers live in an unreal world. In many ways they are like grown-up schoolboys, still being told what to do. They operate on a strict routine which is largely driven by a coach and a football club that have very definite expectations and requirements. Everything is timed to the minute. At every appointment there is a dress code, and your obligations are clear. You don't even have to buy your own clothes. Just about everything you have to wear is supplied. The coach and the club, and the enormous support network is in place to look after your every need. Your only responsibility is to turn up on time every time, ready to do what you are paid handsomely to do.

I suspect it's the same for most professional sportsmen in a team environment. The guidelines are rigid and strict. In lots of ways this is great. Especially the way the Brisbane Lions chose to play their football from that unforgettable turning point at Carlton in 2001, when we became a triple premiership team in the making.

Football teaches you discipline and teamwork: how to be reliable, and how to rely on others. How to understand, accept and appreciate your individual role within a bigger structure, and the importance of doing what is expected of you. It's a winning formula in football, and it has just as much importance in business and everyday life.

Being a professional sportsman was, for me, a dream come true. I count myself extraordinarily fortunate to have been very well paid to pursue something I loved for 17 years. And to receive VIP treatment throughout the journey. I had the best support network in the business in the last few years of my career.

Don't for one moment think it's a cushy job, though. It's not. It's a seven-day-a-week business during the competition phase, from February to September, after a pre-season from November to January in which you train six days a week, often twice a day. You get eight weeks' holiday a year — if you are lucky — and you need it.

Football is about extremes: the extremely good and the extremely bad. You enjoy opportunities you would never get in normal everyday life, but at times you pay a very high price. The focus on professional footballers is massive. There aren't too many other jobs in which, if you have a bad day at the office, it's plastered all over the papers, the television and the radio, and everyone wants to talk about it. Even your fondest supporters will occasionally take the opportunity to remind you of their lofty expectations if you've not done well. You can't leave your work at work.

It's not as if you're breaking rocks every hour of the day at work, and sometimes work might be lying on a portable table getting a massage, but it's still a time commitment. It has some pluses: sometimes on a Wednesday morning we could sneak in a game of golf although the last few years, the management of injuries dictated that I spent more time at the physio instead. Often I was available to drop Madison at school and Tom at kindy in the morning. But a night away with the family is out of the question.

I wasn't long into retirement when I realised that I was missing my daily interaction with the playing group. We'd been together for such a long time and it was such a big part of my life — it's been a big change. I compensate a little by getting out for an occasional game of golf with a few of the boys.

I still like training and getting to the gym two or three days a week, and I even go for a run occasionally. After so many problems getting fit enough to return to football, I've learned never to take my health for granted, so I will never quit exercise altogether. But I must admit that when I wake up on those days when I just don't feel like hitting the gym — I think we all have these days! — it's good not to have to worry about letting anyone down. I can just roll over and go back to sleep.

I've become a good football-watcher, which is more than I could say during my playing days. I used to hate watching because it meant I wasn't playing. In 1995, when I only played one game, one of the toughest times each week was game time. The opportunity to be involved with the media on game days has been enjoyable and has helped make my transition from player to ex-player fairly stress-free. I love watching the progress of the younger players I used to play with and against, and I'm fortunate that the Lions have involved me in a minor way, helping the young forwards at training once a week.

When I became ill I had to focus on life after football — at an age when most players, if they've settled comfortably enough into an AFL career, are just looking forward to the good times and not giving it a thought. This was fortunate, really. I knew my career could end at any moment and I had to be prepared.

Modern players are lucky in that AFL clubs, the AFL and the AFL Players' Association (AFLPA) all devote a massive amount of time and energy to educating players in non-football areas. It wasn't so necessary when I began in 1988, because in those days every player also had a full-time job. At times we'd train in the morning before work and again in the evening after work. There was no extra guidance on how to conduct yourself with the media, or any extra education. You just felt your way, and followed the example of the senior players. That's where I was lucky at Fitzroy, having blokes like Paul Roos, Gary Pert and Matty Rendell around.

I consider myself fortunate because I was ready for life after football. Certainly, my illness-induced mid-career refocus helped significantly, but in the last couple of years I also spent quite a bit of time preparing for the next phase of my life. I was ready for it, and, most importantly, I was excited about it.

I was surprised how busy I was in the first six months of retirement. So much so that a very important lesson was reinforced: I still have to be careful of my CFS. Going around madly for a few months, trying to get all sorts of things in order, I got badly run down. The headaches returned. It was a timely wake-up call.

The first post-football job opportunity that went by the wayside was breakfast radio. I had a chance to join the Triple M breakfast crew in Brisbane, attending to all sporting matters from 5am till 9am. It would have been sensational for an all-sports fanatic like me, and for a few weeks I fantasised about doing it. Opportunities like that don't come along very often. But one night when I must have looked worse than normal, Peta said to me, 'You're not seriously thinking about doing it, are you?' She was right. My health just wouldn't cope. I'd got myself run down just by going at things pretty hard during normal working hours. Getting up at 4am five days a week was out of the question.

Happily, I was still able to join the Triple M football team which took on a three-year commitment to call all Brisbane Lions games. I'm an expert comments man commenting on some of my best mates. That'll take a bit of getting used to, but not nearly as much as the transition from 'we' (as in Lions) to 'they'.

After three years as a player contracted to Fox Footy for endorsement purposes and appearances I was also fortunate to be able to continue that association: there will be more commentary and one-off specials. I'm also writing a newspaper column for *The Sunday Mail* in Brisbane and the Hobart *Mercury*. Doing them is a great way to stay involved in football and talk about the thing I know most about.

I've always enjoyed the media, and I like to think I've had a reasonably good relationship with most journalists and reporters. At times, like anyone, I was a bit sensitive to what they wrote or said, especially in the early days, but the older and wiser I got the more I realised that most of them were pretty fair and reasonable, and they were only doing their job.

My belief is that just like everything in a team environment, you have to share the load. If everyone does their bit, the burden on any one player is never too great.

I was never one to collect newspaper clippings or anything like that but Mum and Peta did a bit of it, and I'm sure that in retirement I'll find a spare moment to look back over the scrapbooks. One thing I know I won't find is more than one or two photographs of Pete. She steadfastly refused throughout most of my career to play the media game. And fair enough — it wasn't her job and she preferred her anonymity. Only once, I think, did she relent — after the 2001 grand final.

I'm also lucky that I've also been employed by the AFL, through AFL Queensland, to do some promotional work. To get out into the community and sell our game, with a strong focus on major junior events and the corporate market. The people at AFLQ, under general manager Richard Griffiths, a former football manager at AFL club Melbourne, are the largely unsung heroes of the success story that is AFL football in Queensland. They do a massive job, building on the success of the Lions and get little recognition.

I'm excited about being able to stay in close contact with football via the media, AFLQ and my minor coaching role, but I'm just as enthusiastic about doing some things outside football.

Simon Skirrow, one-time global vice-president of Adidas, approached me to help him develop a new range of football boots in January 2004. Among Simon's various claims to fame was that he designed, in conjunction with former Australian and Liverpool soccer star Craig Johnston, the world-renowned soccer boot known as the Predator. Simon and his family have now settled in Brisbane.

It's been a fantastic experience and I was really proud when the boots hit the shelves of sporting goods and other retail stores across Australia, the United Kingdom and the United States in March 2005. They go under the brand name Nomis.

They are among the lightest boots on the market, and are made of kangaroo leather which has been treated in such a way that when it gets wet it doesn't get slippery. Rather, it gets more grippy. So instead of a wet ball sliding off the side of a player's boot, the ball is much more likely to go straight because the boot offers a much better purchase on it. I wish they'd been around in my day!

Simon and I spoke on the phone a couple of times; our first face-to-face meeting was on the golf course. I took Lions teammate Chris Scott along for company and we played at North Lakes Golf Course, about 30 minutes' drive north of Brisbane. It was a drizzly day which just got worse, and we were forced to walk off the course at the end of the 10th hole. It must have been very wet, because Scotty was one under par at that stage and even he didn't protest.

Sitting in the clubhouse watching the rain falling we got talking about Simon's idea and his leather which didn't get slippery when it got wet. The first thing I said to him was, 'Well you'd better make a golf glove as well.' So we did. They hit the market in Australia and the United Kingdom in late 2004.

Simon wanted some advice on what an athlete needed from a pair of football boots, so I became something of a research consultant. We took advice from the club podiatrist and physiotherapists and, most importantly, from players. Bit by bit we fine-tuned what was required, and in the end we came up with a product which I genuinely believe is the best boot on the market. I hope I'm right, because my role is to get it on the feet of as many elite players as possible, and to get it into shops Australia-wide.

In my 17 years in football, my team finished in the top four six times, the bottom four six times, and in the middle bracket five times. As well as the three premierships there was a wooden spoon in 1998 and almost another in 1991. I experienced the good times and the bad, and everything in between. And like everyone, in the twilight years of my career I wished I'd known at 17 what I knew at 35.

So rather than being one of those ex-players who thinks they know more than the current players, I want to be one who actually helps the current players, particularly the younger ones, through what can be a difficult journey. I'm having a crack at athlete management — not just of AFL players, but also of people in other codes and other sports.

No matter what sport it is, particularly team sport, the principles are the same. Look, listen and learn in the early days, and don't speak too much except when you are spoken to. You have to try to be quiet yet quietly confident, modest yet self-assured, respectful of the senior players yet not in awe of them.

So I'm now a media commentator, coach, sporting-goods developer and marketer, guest speaker, and an athlete manager in the making, I hope.

But first and foremost, as I look forward to life after football, I'm a husband and a father. That's the most important thing to me. It's the motivation for wanting to be successful in all the other things. I want to be able to provide a quality lifestyle and quality opportunities for my family. For 17 years it was about me. Now it's about us.

I really cherish the time I spend with Madison, Tom and Claudia. I was 29 when I became a father — a pretty good age, I think, because I was old enough to appreciate the joy and responsibility of bringing into the world someone who was actually part of me. I've enjoyed watching them grow up and enjoyed a hands-on role in parenthood. I've changed a few nappies in my time, but my specialties are pick-ups and drop-offs. I've forgotten once or twice, but I haven't lost anyone yet.

I've also enjoyed starting to repay a massive debt to my wife Peta. It'll take me a lifetime, and even that may not be long enough. Because without her I would never have experienced the ultimate joys of my chosen sport. I would have retired in 1995, a frustrated 27-year-old who had played 134 AFL games and never tasted the thrill of finals football. I would have succumbed to the multitude of pressures and frustrations of CFS. Pete, more than anyone else, convinced me not to let it beat me, and to keep going when at times it would have been easier to give it away. She gave me all the support I needed to get through the bad times, and together we enjoyed the good times. All the way to 306 games, 20 finals and three premierships.

I'm still careful with my health, and I always will be. I've learned that you have to be when you've had CFS. Though I feel I've conquered it, I've also learned never to get complacent. That's when it will sting the hardest.

Do I wish I hadn't gone to Cairns in 1994? I don't really know. I know I could have lived without the CFS, but I may have got sick anyway. And if I hadn't got sick I might not have still been playing football through the

Brisbane Lions' golden era. It was an impossible dream come true — and an incredible journey.

I've learned many things along the way, but perhaps the biggest lesson of all is never to take your health for granted. It's much, much too precious. Without your health, all the other things in the world are meaningless. While I thought I'd never admit this, I now believe that I am a better person for the experience of CFS. A better father and a better husband. Because I've learned to appreciate the important things in life, like family and friends. And good health. Never again will I take it for granted and hopefully my experiences can reinforce for CFS sufferers that although at times you feel like its an endless tunnel of frustration and uncertainty, there can and will be life after CFS. And if even one person can get better or be better through having read about my experiences, this book has all been worthwhile.

ALASTAIR LYNCH

AT A GLANCE

Date of Birth: 19 June 1968
Place of Birth: Burnie (Tasmania)
Family Status: Married to Peta with three children —
Madison (born 19 September 1997), Tom (born 18 May
2000) and Claudia (born 24 July 2003)
AFL career: 1988–2004
AFL games: 306; AFL finals: 20
AFL goals: 633; AFL finals goals: 65

Originally from Wynyard, he played senior football with
Hobart in 1986–87 and was drafted from Hobart at No. 50 in
the first AFL national draft in 1986. He played 120 games
with Fitzroy (1988–1993) and 186 games with Brisbane
Bears/Lions (1994–2004).

FOOTBALL HONOURS

Member Brisbane Lions premiership sides 2001, 2002, 2003
Member Brisbane Lions grand final side 2004
Member Brisbane Lions Ansett Cup grand final side 2001
Member Fitzroy's Foster's Cup grand final side 1992

All-Australian selection 1993
AFL Mark of the Year 1989

Four top 10 B&F finishes Fitzroy — 6th 1990, R/Up 1991,
3rd 1992, Winner 1993
Six top 10 B&F finishes Brisbane Bears/Lions — 8th 1994,
10th 1996, 10th 1997, 5th 1998, 9th 2000, 10th 2001

Fitzroy leading goal-kicker 1993
Brisbane Bears leading goal-kicker 1996, No. 2 LGK 1994
Brisbane Lions leading goal-kicker 2000, 2001, 2002, 2003,
No. 2 LGK 2004, No. 3 LGK 1999

Six top 10 finishes in AFL goal-kicking — 7th 1993,
9th 1996, 4th 2000, 2nd 2001, 2nd 2002, 2nd 2003

Tasmanian State of Origin representative
1988–89–90–91–92–93 (deputy vice-captain 1993)

Fitzroy vice-captain 1991–92–93
Brisbane Bears vice-captain 1994–95–96
Brisbane Lions co-captain 1997–98–99–00

Member Fitzroy Team of Fifty Years (1944–1993)
Member Fitzroy Team of the Century (1897–1996)
Member Tasmanian Team of the Century (1905–2004)
Brisbane Lions life member 1997

In 2004 he became the 23rd player to kick 600 AFL goals, and the 43rd player to play 300 AFL games. He also ranked equal 5th in all-time AFL finals goals at the end of his career.

A 'Living Legend' of Tasmanian football, he was further recognised in 2004 when the state's highest individual award, formerly the William Leitch Medal, was renamed the Alastair Lynch Medal in recognition of his achievement in becoming the first Tasmanian to play 300 AFL games.

AFL CAREER SUMMARY

	AFL Games	AFL Goals	AFL Finals	Ladder Position	B&F Placing	Brownlow Votes	Coach
1988	18	24	0	12/14	14th	0	David Parkin
1989	18	26	0	6/14	27th	1	Rod Austin
1990	22	19	0	12/14	6th	0	Rod Austin
1991	22	9	0	14/15	2nd	4	Robert Shaw
1992	20	27	0	10/15	T3rd	2	Robert Shaw
1993	20	68	0	11/15	1st	10	Robert Shaw
1994	13	35	0	12/15	8th	7	Robert Walls
1995	1	2	0	8/16	N/A	0	Robert Walls
1996	18	52	3	3/16	10th	2	John Northey
1997	20	12	1	8/16	10th	0	John Northey
1998	15	10	0	16/16	5th	0	John Northey & Roger Merrett
1999	17	31	3	4/16	21st	0	Leigh Matthews
2000	22	68	2	5/16	9th	3	Leigh Matthews
2001	23	58	2	1/16	11th	3	Leigh Matthews
2002	22	74	3	1/16	15th	4	Leigh Matthews
2003	22	78	4	1/16	8th	5	Leigh Matthews
2004	13	40	2	2/16	22nd	2	Leigh Matthews
Total	306	633	20	–	–	43	
Fitzroy	120	173	0				
Brisbane	186	460	20				

PETER BLUCHER is a well-respected sports journalist and author who, as long-serving communications manager of the Brisbane Lions and a close friend of Alastair Lynch, witnessed first-hand the great player's battle with chronic fatigue. Yet even he was astonished by some of the revelations in a tale that is truly a triumph of spirit over adversity.